EQUITABLE SOLUTIONS FOR RETAINING A ROBUST STEM WORKFORCE: BEYOND BEST PRACTICES

EQUITABLE SOLUTIONS FOR RETAINING A ROBUST STEM WORKFORCE: BEYOND BEST PRACTICES

Donna Joyce Dean, Ph.D.

and

Janet Bandows Koster, MBA, CAE

ELSEVIER

AMSTERDAM • BOSTON • HEIDELBERG • LONDON
NEW YORK • OXFORD • PARIS • SAN DIEGO
SAN FRANCISCO • SINGAPORE • SYDNEY • TOKYO

Academic Press is an imprint of Elsevier

Academic Press is an imprint of Elsevier
32 Jamestown Road, London NW1 7BY, UK
225 Wyman Street, Waltham, MA 02451, USA
525 B Street, Suite 1800, San Diego, CA 92101-4495, USA

Notice
No responsibility is assumed by the publisher for any injury and/or damage to persons
or property as a matter of products liability, negligence or otherwise, or from any use or
operation of any methods, products, instructions or ideas contained in the material herein.
Because of rapid advances in the medical sciences, in particular, independent verification of
diagnoses and drug dosages should be made

British Library Cataloguing-in-Publication Data
A catalogue record for this book is available from the British Library

Library of Congress Cataloging-in-Publication Data
A catalog record for this book is available from the Library of Congress

ISBN: 978-0-12-800215-5

For information on all Academic Press publications
visit our website at elsevierdirect.com

Typeset by TNQ Books and Journals
www.tnq.co.in

Printed and bound by CPI Group (UK) Ltd, Croydon, CR0 4YY

14 15 16 17   10 9 8 7 6 5 4 3 2 1

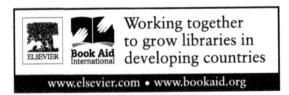

Contents

PART 1
SURVEYING THE LANDSCAPE

PART 2
AWARD-WINNING SOLUTIONS

PART 3
ADVANCING COMPREHENSIVE SOLUTIONS

Foreword

Few will argue that including a broad cross-section of talented people in the scientific research community is not only fair, but also advantageous. A particular example, which is also the focus of this book, is the importance of including women researchers in the STEM fields. However, a number of complex cultural, social, and economic forces within this community and beyond can make inclusion and retention of women, and some men, challenging. Among these challenges is the nature of the workplace at academic institutions, which often conflicts with life outside academia. While changing the academic research culture to reduce or eliminate these conflicts may be the ultimate goal, the means to get from "here" to "there" may not be simple or quick.

Equitable Solutions for Retaining a Robust STEM Workforce: Beyond Best Practices aims to support movement in that direction by providing case studies of projects developed to address a variety of work/life challenges. From supporting travel for dual-career couples to making strategic choices around work/life issues to overcoming implicit bias, these case studies provide detailed examples of ideas in action, discussing how they were implemented, what worked and what did not work, and conclusions that may be drawn from these initiatives. Readers may find programs they wish to imitate, ideas they like but need to modify, and/or the motivation to begin or continue their own efforts.

Taken together, these ideas reinforce the reality that while the need for cultural change in this area is widespread, the actual transformation is likely to come not from a single, sweeping declaration, but from the collective impact of many initiatives, such as those described in this book. In this way, experimental efforts can become recognized best practices, which ultimately become the new norms—in the academic world and beyond.

In gathering these examples, the authors and AWIS are doing us all a great service, not only by collecting in one volume new ideas we can implement at our own institutions, but also by implicitly challenging those who are not already engaged in this kind of work. These recent successes say: If others can do it and achieve great benefits, why not you?

Patrick Farrell, PhD
Provost and Vice President for Academic Affairs
Lehigh University
September 2013

Preface

In March 2012, the Association of Women in Science assembled a group of experts in New York City for a workshop on "Rethinking the Future of the STEM Workplace: Convening of Global Experts on Work/Life Family Issues." The workshop discussed programs, best practices and, ultimately, solutions for retaining a competitive and innovative scientific workforce. The presenters were grant recipients from the Elsevier Foundation New Scholars Program. Established in 2006, the New Scholars Program addresses the attrition rate of talented women scientists caused by work/life integration issues and advances innovative approaches to creating a more family friendly workplace. Recognizing that all women scientists must traverse the path through academia as part of their training, the program has focused on fostering a more equitable academia by supporting projects likely to make significant impacts on these institutions so that early- to midcareer women scientists may successfully integrate family responsibilities with demanding careers. Key aspects of the program include (1) encouraging networking and collaborations among institutions and/or across the science, technology, engineering, and mathematics (STEM) disciplines in ways that support the challenges of faculty and staff with family responsibilities; (2) developing and implementing strategies for advocacy and policy development that advance knowledge and awareness and foster the adoption of programs to recruit, retain, and develop women in science; and (3) enabling scientists to attend conferences, meetings, workshops, and symposia that are critical to their career development by helping them fulfill child care and other family responsibilities when attending such gatherings. Recent grants have thus promoted institutional research, advocacy, and policy development to retain, recruit, and develop women in science and have enabled researchers to attend conferences critical to their careers by assisting with child care, mentorship, and networking.

In light of these objectives, the workshop provided a framework in which grantees could learn from one other. Participants shared lessons learned from developing and implementing their projects and discussed the hurdles they faced. They also discussed extensively the tactics they used in overcoming these hurdles, along with plans for sustaining their programs beyond the terms of the grant.

The event's anticipated outcomes were as follows:

- A fuller understanding of the emerging and pressing concerns of today's Global STEM workforce regarding work/life effectiveness and the advancement of working women.

- A collection of recommendations from thought leaders and practitioners who are leading efforts in work/life effectiveness, diversity, and workplace equity about the tools, resources, and policy changes needed.
- Creation of a report distilled from these recommendations that is intended to serve as an action plan to help employers, working women, and policy makers identify, create, and sustain systemic changes.
- Collaborations to form plans to stem the attrition of talented women from the academic pipeline. The plans' objectives are to provide institutions with the tools they need to help retain women in academia as well as to develop policies that will catalyze the transformation of the international STEM workforce.

Finding the appropriate balance between work and life is a challenge for both male and female scientists and, increasingly, also concerns (to widely varying degrees) the universities, businesses, and other organizations that employ them. As an eminent publisher of scientific, technical, and medical information products and services, Elsevier has distinguished itself as a leader in fostering policy change to accommodate the new realities of the twenty-first-century STEM workplace. By seeding the development of unique approaches that allow early- to midcareer women scientists to balance family responsibilities with demanding careers, the lessons learned from Elsevier's New Scholars Program grant recipients can help define and shape the STEM workplaces and workforces of tomorrow.

Our hope is that this book can provide academic institutions with the tools they need to help retain women along every step of the career pathway. We also envision it as a catalyst for the development of government policies that work for positive transformation of the STEM workforce in all work sectors. The talented individuals pursuing STEM careers across the globe deserve workplaces that recognize and accommodate both their dedication to their professions and their humanity.

Donna Joyce Dean
Janet Bandows Koster

October 2013
Alexandria, VA

Acknowledgments

We are indebted to the many individuals who contributed significant insights and critical support for this undertaking. Specifically, we wish to thank:

The featured Elsevier Foundation New Scholars awardees, for their lively participation at the global roundtable in March 2012 that formed the foundation of this book: Michele Garfinkel, Joan Girgus, Theodore Hodapp, Mary Anne Holmes, George Kamkamidze, Christine Littleton, Sandra Masur, Angela Doyle McNerney, Elizabeth Pollitzer, Maria Santore, Barbara Silver, Cindy Simpson, and Gerlind Wallon.

Susan Fitzpatrick, Joan S. Herbers, and Kelly Mack, for providing excellent leadership at the roundtable discussions.

Adrian Mulligan and Gemma Deakin of Elsevier Research and Academic Relations, for their phenomenal efforts in data acquisition and analysis of global work/life patterns. The results they delivered provide unparalleled quantitative support for the work/life concepts presented here; without them, there would have been no Chapter 2.

Sophia Huyer of Women in Global Science and Technology and Elizabeth Pollitzer of Portia Ltd, for graciously sharing their extensive knowledge on global approaches to policy development and for contributing significant portions of Chapter 9.

Erin Cadwalader, the Phoebe S. Leboy Public Policy Fellow for the Association for Women in Science, for contributing Chapter 8—an excellent homage to the efforts of Dr Leboy and to her legacy.

Mary Preap, Associate Acquisitions Editor of Academic Press/Elsevier, who made the process of book publication painless and efficient.

Miranda Spencer, for her insightful questioning and careful technical editing, which significantly improved the book's content.

David Ruth, Senior Vice President of Global Communications and Executive Director of the Elsevier Foundation, and Ylann Schemm, Program Manager of the Elsevier New Scholars Program, for their extraordinary vision in developing and supporting a grant program that rewards new and innovative approaches. They have leveraged changes in global workplaces that exceed by orders of magnitude their initial financial investment.

PART 1

Surveying the Landscape

Envisioning the STEM Workplace of the Future: The Need for Work/Life Programs and Family-Friendly Practices

I am discovering something new for my academic field. —**A woman working in engineering and technology, age 26–35 years, single, Turkey**

Life is short; stretching myself to the limit will only lead to burnout. I am not going to commit myself to low-priority projects, even if I have to forego recognition and promotion. —**A woman working in medicine and allied health, age 46–55 years, married/partnered, Malaysia**

The body of basic and empirical research on work/life issues is vast. Governments, corporations, universities, and professional societies across many disciplines and around the globe have taken surveys, issued white papers, and published articles in peer-reviewed journals. Lists of best practices recommendations ranging from flexible workplace structures to onsite child care centers abound. Laws are in place; the United States has Title IX, which bans sex discrimination in education and in government-funded programs, and countries across the Eurozone operate under a plethora of family-friendly policies supported by the State. Some nations have even introduced gender-based quotas. Yet data about successful programs and the implementation strategies associated with them are very limited.

This book is designed to remedy that disparity.

A COMMON DEFINITION OF WORK/LIFE BALANCE

Balance, satisfaction, integration, and *flexibility* are some of the many terms associated with modern societies' tug-of-war between the demands of the workplace and workers' private lives. Reaching an acceptable level of accommodation between the two has become not only an individual determination but also a systemic debate among employers across all science, technology, engineering, and mathematics (STEM) sectors around the globe.

The good news is that both men and women in increasingly equal numbers are seeking an acceptable balance. In fact, evidence from the survey by the Association of Women in Science (discussed more fully in Chapter 2) points to notable differences between the oldest and youngest age cohorts, particularly with regard to the job flexibility they enjoy. Fully 45% of those under age 36 years said that they plan to move— many abroad—for the sake of their career. Despite the current funding climate for research, younger employees do not feel they have to remain loyal to one employer. They will go wherever they think will further their careers and, increasingly, wherever will enable them to work in the way that they want, allowing them to juggle their various interests and responsibilities.

THE CURRENT CLIMATE

As will be discussed in Chapters 3 and 4, an increasing number of companies and institutions worldwide are faced with the challenge of recruiting and managing employees who are part of a dual-career couple. Some work sectors and specific disciplines have begun to grapple with this issue. A particularly cogent example is the recent effort by the petroleum engineering community to assess its workforce demographics. With more than 46,000 members worldwide, the Society of Petroleum Engineers represents a workforce employed largely in national and international companies rather than in the academic or government sectors. In a May 2011 survey of its members in 93 countries, the organization discovered that dual-career couples comprise about half of the petroleum engineering workforce. Two significant challenges for these families are child rearing and relocation.[1,2] A second survey in December 2011, designed to obtain a more comprehensive view of employment issues that will face the industry over the next few decades, focused on those under age 45 years.[3] The data show very clearly that within the next two decades, a large fraction of the petroleum industry workforce will be female and that those women will be part of a dual-career couple. This trend is summarized in the organization's report on the two surveys:

> Polices on relocation, flexible hours, and telecommuting should be reviewed to determine whether more dual-career friendly policies can be implemented. The issue is not how we have traditionally done business and acquired critical experiences and skills but rather what must get done and how it can be done with a workforce that has different domestic responsibilities than the vanishing workforce that was dominated by a single breadwinner. In the past, companies benefitted from having employees with non-working spouses, who serve[d] as full time domestic personal assistants. That fraction of the workforce is now rapidly shrinking.

The petroleum engineering community is not unique in recognizing the changing demographics of STEM professions and the need for the workplace to reflect them. Women now earn approximately half of all US MD degrees and PhD degrees in biomedical disciplines, but their success in educational attainments does not run parallel to their success in employment. In academia, women hold relatively few of the senior professorships in medical schools or senior research positions at corporations employing biomedical scientists. In medical schools, this trend can be attributed to too few women entering or remaining in the assistant professor positions that are the springboards to senior faculty positions. Meanwhile, the proportion of female PhDs in the availability pool for biomedical science careers (47%) is almost twice that for the physical sciences (26%). Yet among assistant professors in top basic science departments, the proportion of women (29%) is little higher than in highly ranked chemistry or physics departments (26% and 25%, respectively). Science department Web sites of very-high-research universities indicate that the proportion of women among entry-level assistant professors usually approximates the gender distribution of recent PhDs in the discipline. In contrast, the proportion of female assistant professors in medical school basic science departments has scarcely budged in recent years, despite a growing PhD pool that is inching over 50%.

Interventions being introduced to solve these problems include establishing more family-friendly policies, providing mentoring, and attempting to modify a climate perceived as unfriendly to women. However, increasing evidence suggests that these "best practices" may not be sufficient to remedy the problem, and that women scientists in academia and at large corporations are discouraged not only by difficulties in attaining professional advancement, but also by long-established structures and standards that place high value on traits perceived as being primarily masculine.

SPURRING SYSTEMIC CHANGE

In this environment, employers who resist tailoring the workplace to retain the best workers of both genders will be increasingly unable to compete in a global marketplace. Many institutions and organizations have begun to recognize this reality. Fortunately, many new ideas are emerging to assist them in that process. The Elsevier New Scholars have created evidence-based programs that address the work/life challenges of STEM employment, including dependent-care responsibilities, dual-career relationships, the need for mentoring, and the ability to travel to professional meetings. The lessons learned from these programs now provide the basis for their broader application in robust and innovative solutions that address the root causes of work/life imbalance in the STEM workplace.

The following chapters provide case studies of successful programs and practical tools that can serve as templates for use by a variety of institutions. They are well researched and can be scaled up and delivered quickly and effectively. All the case studies share a common structure outlining the functional stages of program implementation: conception, exploration, implementation, evaluation, and sustainability. When considering the programs they describe for application in one's own workplace, it is important to remember that these stages are not linear, as each impacts the others in complex ways. For example, considering sustainability factors is very much a part of the exploration process, and implementation methods directly affect sustainability. In other cases, an organization might need to hold off from implementation to explore better options based on new information about changing demographics.

Finally, each chapter closes with practical tools that can be used by any institution to develop programs similar to those described in the case studies.

2

Work/Life Integration Challenges Are Worldwide

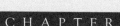

I'm willing to relocate most anywhere for a permanent position. **—A man working in physics, age 26–35 years, married/partnered, Germany**

During my doctoral program, I felt pressured to perform and that negatively impacted my overall happiness. Now that I have reduced my focus on work, I have felt happier at home, which has improved my productivity at work. **—A man working in social sciences, age 46–55 years, married/partnered, Canada**

Work/life integration issues are having demonstrable impacts on the science, technology, engineering, and mathematics (STEM) workforce. In the largest survey ever undertaken of work/life integration issues among publishing scientists, Association of Women in Science (AWIS), with funding from the Elsevier Foundation, collected information on the topic from scientists and researchers worldwide. Summary results from the survey were released during the 2012 "Rethinking the Future of the STEM Workplace" conference sponsored by AWIS and the foundation in New York to coincide with International Women's Day and the United Nation's

56th session of the Commission on the Status of Women[4] (see Appendices A and B).

The survey's findings raised serious concerns about retaining scientific talent, sustaining innovation within the current science workplace, and keeping both women and men engaged in research endeavors. The data showed that key factors including lack of flexibility in the workplace, dissatisfaction with career development opportunities, and low salaries are driving both men and women to reconsider their profession. The first detailed overview of the analyzed data is presented in this chapter.

SURVEY METHODS AND DATA ANALYSIS

Between December 2011 and January 2012, a total of 51,380 individuals were randomly selected from across 1.2 million international authors who had published in 2009.[5] These authors were sent via e-mail an invitation to participate in the "Research Insights Index" survey, which included 15 questions on work/life issues plus demographic questions (see Appendix C). The online survey took approximately 12–15 min to complete. When the survey closed on January 31, 2012, a total of 4225 scientists had responded, equal to a response rate of 9.5% (in proportion to the valid base of 44,351 individuals, from which 7029 individuals were excluded because the e-mails were returned undeliverable). In order to ensure proportional representation by country and discipline, mailings were controlled. That is, if response was low from a certain group, then additional invitations were sent. Because representativeness was achieved via this managed mailing strategy, the data were not weighted. Results at the top level are based on 4225 responses and have a margin of error that is ±1.3% at the 90% confidence level.

As shown in Figure 2.1, 36% of respondents were from Western Europe (including 6% from the United Kingdom, 6% from Italy, 5% from Germany, 3% from Spain, and 3% from France). Twenty-eight percent were from North America (24% from the United States and 4% from Canada). Twenty-two percent were from Asia Pacific (APAC, including 6% from China and 4% from Japan). Six percent were from Latin America, and 6% were from Eastern Europe. The remaining 2% were from Africa and the Middle East. Highlights of findings from specific countries are included, along with broader regional analyses in the subsequent figures in this chapter. Worldwide, not surprisingly, older respondents had more published articles than did younger respondents.

Of the 4225 respondents, 64% worked at a university, not surprising given that academic scientists tend to publish more research papers than those in other employment sectors (See Figure 2.2). Eighty-three percent

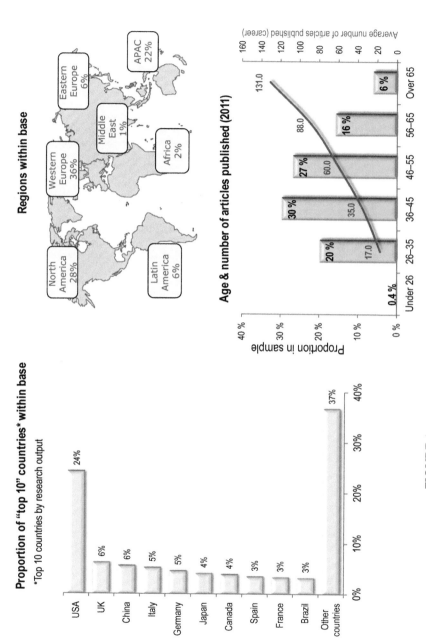

FIGURE 2.1 Country, region, and age of survey respondents.

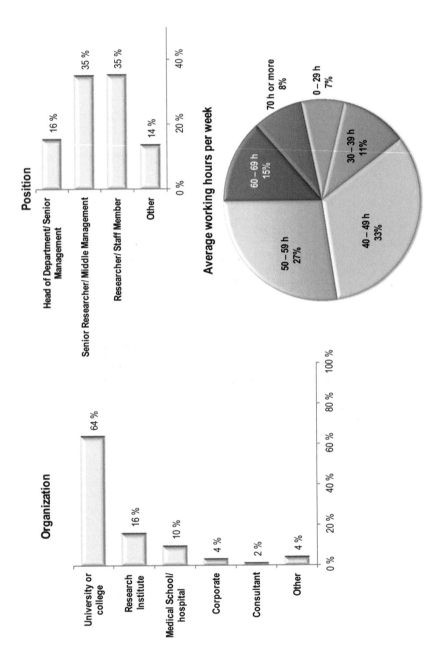

FIGURE 2.2   Job role and organization of survey respondents.

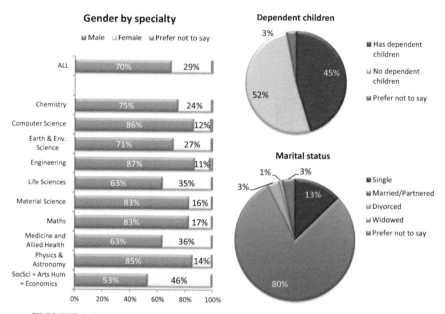

FIGURE 2.3   Gender and relationship or family status of survey respondents.

reported that they worked 40 or more hours per week. Almost three-quarters were researchers or worked at middle-management levels.

Eighty percent of the respondents were married or partnered and 70% were male, as detailed in Figure 2.3. The gender distribution was not surprising, given the global scope of the survey and historical patterns of career progression in the STEM disciplines. These individuals published academically across a broad range of disciplines. For purpose of analysis, the data were grouped into nine fields of endeavor: chemistry, computer science, earth and environmental science, engineering, life sciences, materials science, mathematics, medicine and allied health, physics and astronomy, plus a tenth category comprising social science, arts/humanities, and economics.

GLOBAL PERSPECTIVES ON CAREERS IN SCIENCE

Of those surveyed, 67% believed that their research was making a difference to society, while 63% were satisfied with their career opportunities (See Figure 2.4). More than half (58%) were happy with their work/life balance. Agreement with the statement that one's research makes a difference to society increased with age, presumably because older researchers have a larger body of work to reflect on than those at an earlier stage in their career. Those in specialties that are more applied and deal directly with people (e.g., medicine) were more likely to report that their research

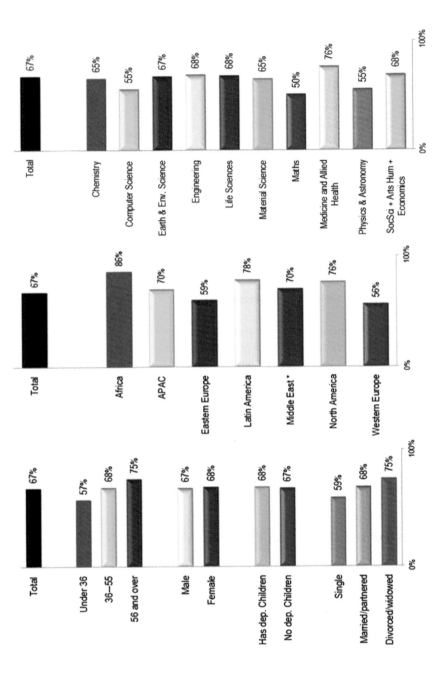

FIGURE 2.4 Percentage of survey respondents who agreed with the statement "I feel like the work I am doing is making a difference to society," analyzed by demographic characteristics, region, and field.

is making a difference than those in more theoretical specialties such as mathematics, physics, and computer science. There was also a difference in opinion by region/country: researchers from Eurozone countries (e.g., Spain, Italy, and Germany) were less likely to agree, perhaps due to funding cuts resulting from the economic crisis there. Agreement was higher in North America and Latin America.

Less than two-thirds of researchers said they are happy with their career opportunities, as shown in Figure 2.5. This percentage did increase with age, from 57% among those under age 36 years to 74% among those aged 56 years and older. Satisfaction was linked to job security (permanent positions), a clear progression path, and having a good work/life balance. Those dissatisfied mentioned lack of a permanent position, low salary, and lack of funding. There were no major differences in response among those in different disciplines, although physicists and astronomers had the lowest level of satisfaction and researchers in medicine and allied health had the highest. Countries in which satisfaction was highest were the United States (66%) and China (74%). Conversely, satisfaction was lowest in European countries, e.g., Italy (46%), Spain (48%), Germany (53%), and the United Kingdom (53%).

Only 58% of those surveyed were happy with their work/life balance. Those who were happy managed to successfully separate their work and personal lives, or were able to reduce their working hours or adopt flexible ones. Those aged 56 years and over were most happy (70%). Only half of the women (52%) reported that they are happy with their work/life integration, compared with 61% of men working in research across all fields. Having dependent children had no impact on these percentages. Fifty-one percent of respondents were single. Researchers in the United Kingdom and Germany were particularly unhappy with their work/life balance.

GENDER DIFFERENCES IN APPROACHES TO WORK/LIFE ISSUES

Being able to say no to nonpriority projects or to delegate tasks and responsibilities provides flexibility and a sense of control over one's time and work efforts. That ability can facilitate necessary choices that must be made between personal life and work life. In the survey, slightly more than half the respondents (53%) agreed that they were comfortable saying no to projects that they did not consider to be a priority. Agreement was less closely linked to seniority than was having others to whom the work could be delegated. A key factor was whether a researcher had a permanent position (tenure) that ensured he or she had more freedom in making decisions. Those disagreeing were not in a position to decide priorities and felt that saying no would damage their careers or their working

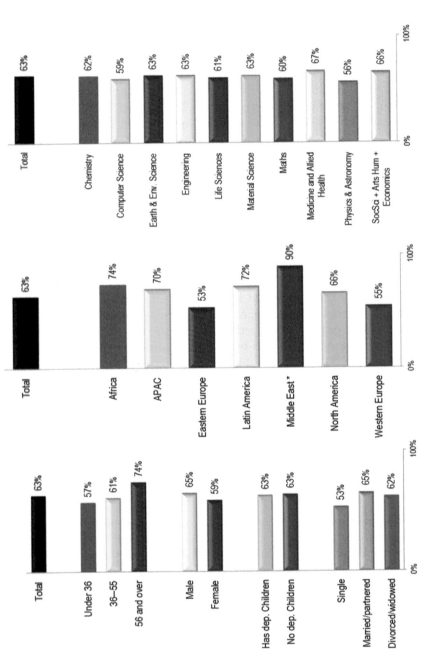

FIGURE 2.5 Percentage of respondents who agreed with the statement "I am satisfied with my career opportunities," analyzed by demographic characteristics, region, and field.

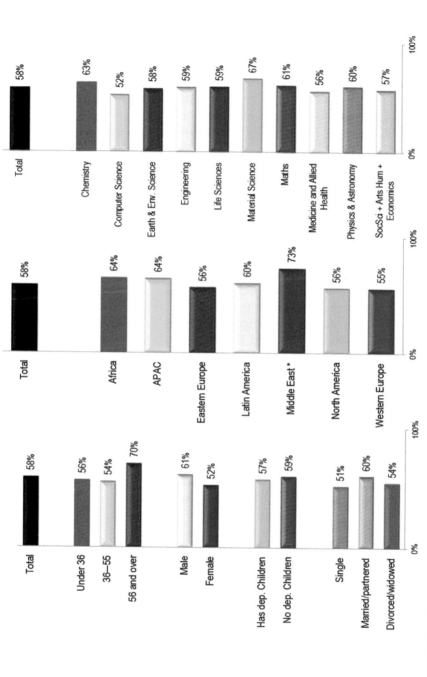

FIGURE 2.6 Percentage of survey respondents who agreed with the statement "I am happy with my work/life balance," analyzed by demographic characteristics, region, and field.

relationship with colleagues. Female researchers were less likely to agree than males (47% compared with 55%). Similarly, agreement increased with age (47% of those under age 36 years agreed versus 65% for those aged 56 years and older). Researchers in North America were more likely to agree (58%) while those in Japan were least likely (29%).

Analysis of survey results revealed that delegation of tasks was a matter of both seniority and gender. Just less than half of researchers (46%) agreed that there were others at work to whom they could delegate tasks. Those agreeing typically had assistants or worked within a team, while those disagreeing did not. Those disagreeing also mentioned that colleagues might not have the specialized knowledge required to undertake certain tasks. Agreement increased with seniority: three-fifths (59%) of department heads agreed compared with 53% of senior researchers and 37% of researchers. Those under age 36 years were less likely to agree (38%), as were female researchers (40%) and those working in the United Kingdom (35%) and Italy (38%). Conversely, researchers aged 36 years and older (48%), male researchers (49%), and those working in Germany (58%) were more likely to agree.

With regard to their personally making efforts to ensure a good work/life balance, one-third of respondents reported that these efforts had negative impacts on their careers, with women (37%) more likely than men (30%) to say this was the case (See Figure 2.9). More than half (51%) of all these scientists and researchers said that work demands conflicted with their personal lives at least two to three times per week. Agreement was higher among those with dependent children (36%) and particularly among female researchers with children (46%) as well as male researchers with children (33%). It was evident from comments in response to open-ended questions that having family commitments limited respondents' ability to relocate for better research positions, and that to be successful in research they had to be focused on their career. Those disagreeing noted there were no negative impacts from having a good work/life balance or said that it enhanced their career performance. Agreement was highest in the United Kingdom (39%), Canada (36%), and China (41%), but lowest in Italy (23%) and Brazil (13%).

GENDER DIFFERENCES AND CAREER/LIFE DECISIONS

Institutional policies can be perceived as family friendly or family unfriendly. As it is not uncommon for researchers to need to relocate for the best research positions, only one-third of researchers surveyed agreed that their institution provided sufficient support for their spouse and were family friendly (See Figure 2.10). Of those agreeing, some reported that their institution had a spousal-hire policy, while others noted that flexible working or benefit plans supported their spouse. Others noted that only

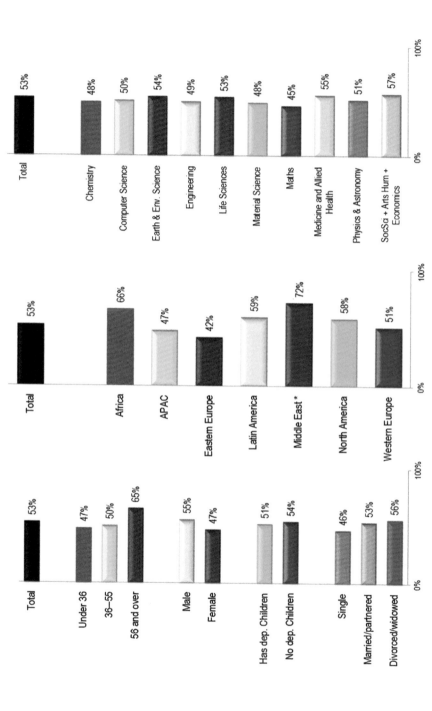

FIGURE 2.7 Percentage of survey respondents who agreed with the statement "I am comfortable saying no to work/projects that I do not consider a priority," analyzed by demographic characteristics, region, and field.

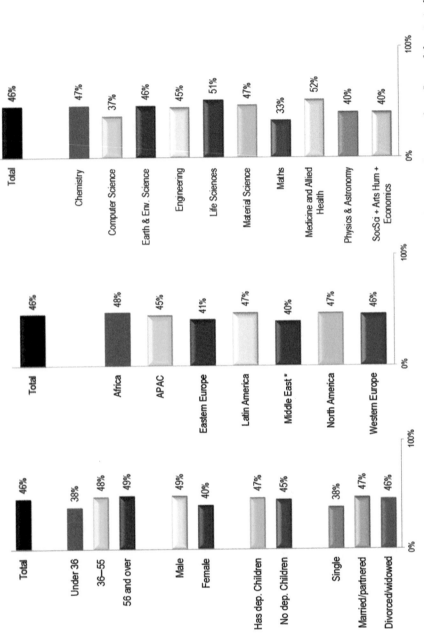

FIGURE 2.8 Percentage of survey respondents who agreed with the statement "At work, there are others to whom I can delegate tasks," analyzed by demographic characteristics, region, and field.

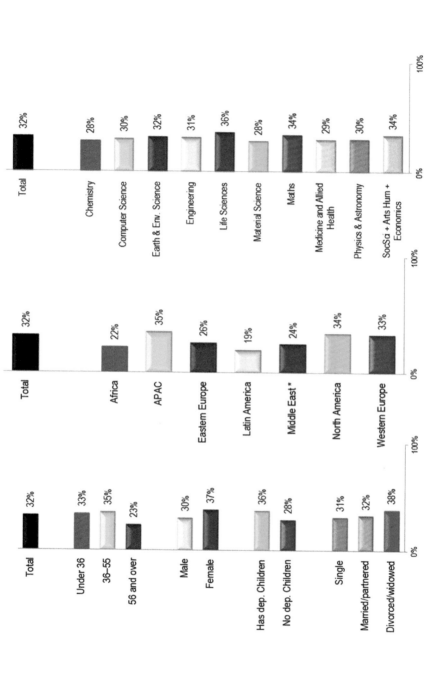

FIGURE 2.9 Percentage of survey respondents who stated that "Ensuring that I have a good work/life balance has negatively impacted my career," analyzed by demographic characteristics, region, and field.

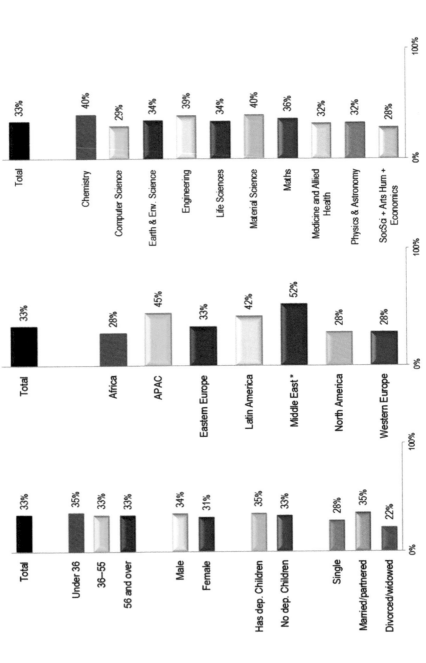

FIGURE 2.10   Percentage of survey respondents reporting that their institutions are family friendly, analyzed by demographic characteristics, region, and field.

low-salaried positions and/or health care support were available to the spouse. Those disagreeing (also 33%) indicated that their institution did not have a spousal-hire policy or that such policies or other types of support were not available because of funding cuts. Agreement was lower than average in North America and Western Europe (28% each), while it was highest in the APAC Region (45%) and Latin America (42%). Only 29% of United States scientists who responded said that their spouse or partner received sufficient support from their institution. By comparison, 65% of Chinese scientists felt that their spouses or partners were receiving sufficient support.

Childbearing was a significant factor for many respondents, as presented in Figure 2.11. Nearly 40% of women respondents said they had delayed having children because of their careers, while 27% of males indicated the same situation. Those agreeing said they were waiting until they had a permanent position or noted that they could not afford to start a family on their current income.

Moving abroad to further their careers was considered by a quarter of respondents (See Figure 2.12). This response was particularly the case for young (45% of those under age 36 years) or single (41%) researchers. Those specializing in sciences such as computer science (38%) and researchers in China (37%) and the Eurozone were more likely to move abroad. Many stated that the expectation of more opportunities, funding, or a permanent position would be motivators for moving abroad. Consideration of this type of career move was notably low in North America (13%).

STRESS AND WORK/LIFE CONFLICTS

Most researchers experienced stress at work and the majority (61%) reported that they have learned to cope with it as summarized in Figure 2.13. Only a small minority (15%) reported that they responded positively to stress, seeing it as an invigorating challenge. Female researchers and those with children were slightly more likely to state that they had learned to cope, as were researchers in Canada (75%), the United Kingdom (70%), and the United States (66%). Italian researchers were the most likely to be invigorated by the challenge (26%). Only 3% of respondents had changed jobs because of stress.

More than half (53%) of all scientists and researchers said that work demands conflicted with their personal lives at least two to three times per week. (See Figures 2.14 and 2.15). This opinion was slightly more common among those with children (61%) and women (58%). As noted above in Figures 2.6, 2.7, and 2.8, even among women without dependent children it was more common. Researchers in the United States (60%), Canada (68%), and the United Kingdom (62%) were most likely to experience a conflict between work and their personal life at least weekly. In the

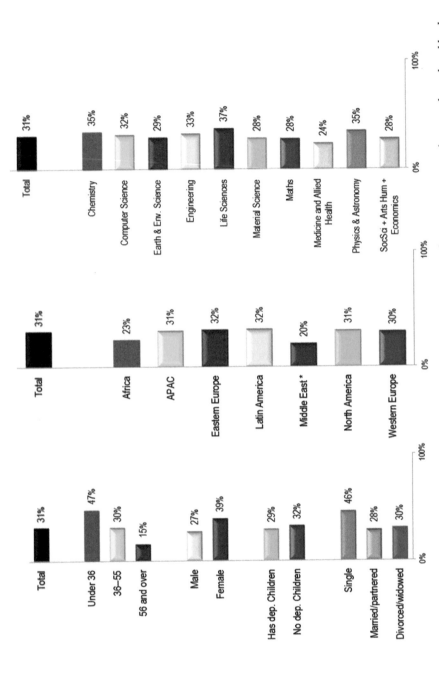

FIGURE 2.11 Percentage of survey respondents who have delayed having children in order to pursue careers in research, analyzed by demographic characteristics, region, and field.

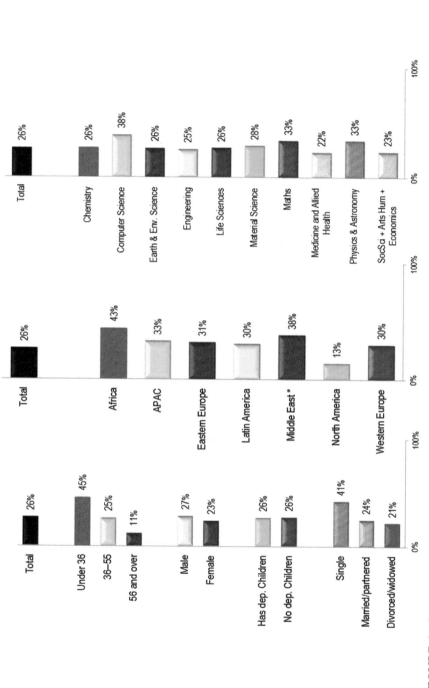

FIGURE 2.12 Percentage of survey respondents who would move to another country to further their careers, analyzed by demographic characteristics, region, and field.

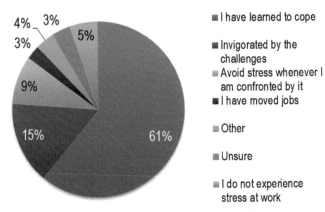

FIGURE 2.13   Attitudes toward stress at work expressed by survey respondents.

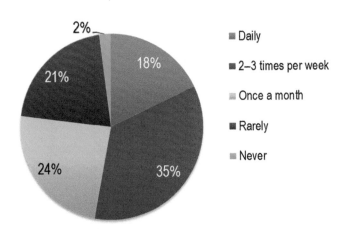

FIGURE 2.14   Survey respondents' reports on how often work demands conflict with personal-life demands.

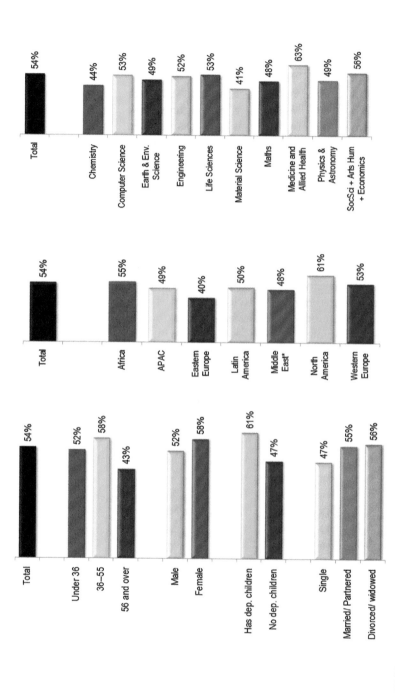

FIGURE 2.15 Demographics of survey respondents who report that work demands conflict with personal-life demands daily or two to three times weekly, analyzed by demographic characteristics, region, and field.

context of discipline, specialists in medicine and allied health professions were the most likely to report a conflict at least weekly (63%).

CAREER MOBILITY AND JOB SECURITY

About half of researchers expected to stay in the same position and a further 16% expected to be promoted (See Figures 2.16 and 2.17). One in 10 expected to leave their current position in the near term, while 13% were uncertain. These expectations varied considerably by age: three-quarters of those aged 56 years and older expected to stay in the same position, and of those expecting to leave, the move was due to retirement. A quarter to a fifth of early-career researchers (under age 36 years) expected to be promoted and a fifth expected to leave their current position. Young researchers expecting to leave were planning to relocate or desired advancement outside their current institution. Only 1 in 10 of those expecting to leave their current position wanted to leave research completely. The other reasons included contracts or funding ending and transitioning to a different career level (e.g., from postdoctoral researcher into a faculty position). Of those intending to leave, women were twice as likely as men to report that their spouse had been offered work elsewhere (12% versus 6%) (See Figure 2.18).

For the approximately 10% of researchers who intended to leave their current position, the reasons given were desire advancement outside the current organization (36%), plan to relocate to another country or city (32%), retirement (11%), leave research and start another career (10%), unable to balance work/life integration (9%), spouse offered work elsewhere (8%), lack of interest in work (7%), or plan to move to a different department in same organization (6%). Many respondents gave multiple reasons, including numerous other reasons cited by 27% of the respondents.

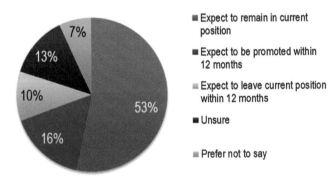

FIGURE 2.16 Survey respondents' near-term perspective regarding their current position.

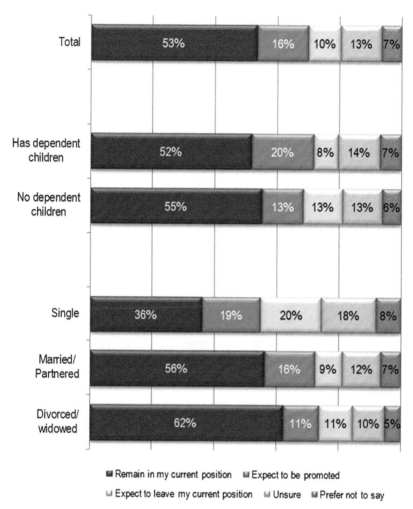

FIGURE 2.17 Relationship and family status of survey respondents and their views on their current positions.

From the data presented here, it is clear that work/life integration presents challenges to scientists. Many individuals observed that their work environments are outmoded and/or that workplace policies are not family friendly. Lack of flexibility in the workplace, dissatisfaction with career development opportunities, and low salaries are driving both men and women to reconsider their professions. These findings have confirmed that work/life conflict is not gender specific in most cases. The real issue is that academic workplaces in particular are still modeled on an ideal that not only no longer exists but also does not complement the realities of today's global workforce.

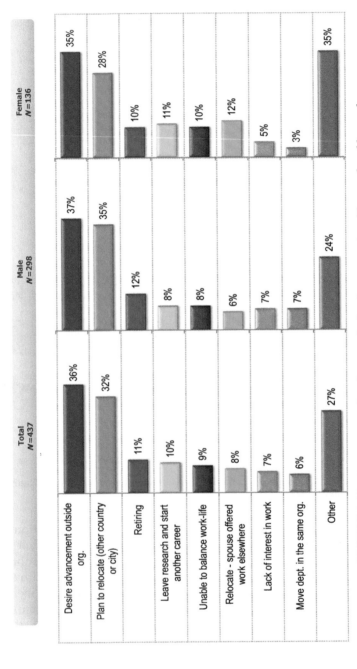

FIGURE 2.18   Survey respondents' reasons for leaving a current position, analyzed by gender.

Award-Winning Solutions

CHAPTER

3

Addressing Work/Life Issues

Equitable Solutions for Retaining a Robust STEM Workforce.
http://dx.doi.org/10.1016/B978-0-12-800215-5.00003-8

31

A good work/life balance is supportive for having good ideas. —A man working in life sciences, age 36–45 years, married/partnered, Germany

True success in research requires publishing at a rate which is not compatible with children and life outside the office. —A woman working in environmental sciences, age 26–35 years, married/partnered, Peru

Significant progress has been made in improving the status of women within the scientific workforce over the past three decades, particularly with regard to training. In many science, technology, engineering, and mathematics (STEM) fields, women have achieved or exceeded parity with men in the number of doctoral degrees received and are well represented in the ranks of postdoctoral researchers. However, at each stage of advancement, from postdoctoral training to first position through progression to higher levels, the proportion of women represented drops off substantially.[6] This exodus has been linked to issues related to their stated inability to establish a satisfactory work and life balance and/or to starting a family.[7] Although many women face the challenge of starting a family just at the time they are hitting stride in their professional career, its impact on women in STEM is especially pronounced—particularly in academia. Women still comprise less than 28% of science and engineering tenured and tenure-track faculty at 4-year colleges and universities.[8] They remain disproportionately represented in the lowest ranks of instructor and lecturer and in unranked positions.

As the survey demonstrated, many of the factors discouraging women (and men) from entering the higher faculty ranks of academia and leadership positions in STEM fields in general are directly related to institutional climate and the challenge of balancing work and home responsibilities. In particular, female faculty members are especially likely to face obstacles related to work/life balance because the academic tenure clock typically coincides with the biologically constrained childbearing and child rearing years of women.

This chapter presents three case studies of Elsevier New Scholars projects that take widely divergent approaches to the "work" and "away from work" conflicts that women scientists may face. All three projects developed pragmatic approaches overcoming these challenges and contain information that should be widely adaptable by scientists in any professional context.

Case study 1 describes the development, modification, and broad applicability of a highly interactive workshop on creating work/life satisfaction that is easily transferrable to any work sector and to any STEM disciplinary context. The participants' workbook and resource guide enable ongoing individual work while the workshop's interactive nature allows participants to share their stories and to learn from each other both during and after the program. Although the program was originally focused solely on women scientists, its content has become highly relevant to male scientists, who face many of the same career-conflict issues. The formulation, pilot testing, and ongoing adaptation, and modification of the program are particularly instructive.

Case study 2 describes a countrywide strategy to provide encouragement and pragmatic information for early career women scientists in an emerging democracy. Subgroups of women with similar scientific backgrounds and interests were identified to whom training sessions were provided on the many elements of an independent scientific career. These sessions were conducted by successful female scientists who could also speak to achieving balance between work and family. A thoughtfully conducted survey of participants enabled the project's leaders to create the most relevant program format and content.

Case study 3 addresses the need to convey the outcomes of research in writing and to prepare cogent proposals for funding research endeavors. While writers in the arts and humanities have long recognized the importance of using retreats to foster consistent writing and greater confidence in one's chosen profession, this approach has not been part of the STEM culture. This case study provides critical information on how to foster a scientific writing retreat that includes coaching on professional writing, peer feedback, blocks of unstructured writing time to improve writing success, and group meals and accommodations to facilitate social connections among participants that can be sustained after the retreat for effective management of work/life issues. This ongoing peer support network is expected to help participants as they face ongoing work/life issues and challenges.

CASE STUDY 1. LEADING WOMEN TO CREATE THEIR OWN DEFINITION OF WORK/LIFE SATISFACTION

Implementing organization: Association for Women in Science, Alexandria, Virginia (2008 Elsevier Foundation New Scholars Grant Awardee).

Project leaders: Cynthia Simpson, MEd, CAE and Janet Bandows Koster, MBA, CAE.

Rationale and Goals

As the only all-inclusive, multidisciplinary organization supporting women in STEM, the Association for Women in Science (AWIS) has a broad membership base, numerous chapters across the country, and close connections with many organizations. AWIS has always promoted a "dual agenda": advocating for improved institutional and departmental policies to support the career advancement of female faculty and empowering women with the resources they need to integrate work and personal life more fully and positively. AWIS believes that universities and academic departments have a primary responsibility to ensure that women have the opportunity to be successful and productive throughout their careers through promotion of policies, development of resources, and fostering of a climate and culture that include zero tolerance for discriminatory comments or behavior.

AWIS supports women in STEM directly by providing programs and resources that help them succeed in managing the demands of family and career, including peer networking, mentoring, and career enhancement programs. In this particular case, AWIS developed and facilitated an educational/support program, "Improving Work-Life Satisfaction", including a "Program-In-A-Box" toolkit with supplementary resources, to provide women in STEM with the tools they need to achieve satisfaction and an effective balance between their professional and personal lives. The first phase of the project was the creation and dissemination of the program to the numerous AWIS chapters around the country.

The AWIS program was designed with the objective of empowering individual women in STEM to (1) examine how their current choices impact work/life balance and identify changes that will have the biggest impact on their personal and professional satisfaction; (2) see personal challenges and opportunities from a fresh perspective; (3) recognize the critical importance of recovering from stressors to stay motivated and engaged; (4) understand how incongruence between values and actions can drain energy; (5) identify and create a plan to eliminate their personal and professional energy drains; and (6) maximize their energy level for improved performance and increased productivity.

Project Description and Outcomes

To understand and then address issues facing women in STEM careers during the development and facilitation of a work/life satisfaction educational/support program, a 20-item survey was sent to 2800 active AWIS members via e-mail. The purpose of this survey was to elicit feedback related to members' work/life balance challenges and the kind of programs that would be most useful to them. The information provided from this survey, combined with additional available research on work/life issues facing women scientists plus the responses from focus groups and chapter pilot programs, allowed AWIS to develop a national pilot program designed to best meet the needs of women in STEM. The pilot program was launched in February 2009 before an audience of 65 women in conjunction with the annual meeting of the American Association for the Advancement of Science (AAAS) in Chicago. Based on participant feedback, content was later refined and program length reduced from 4 to 2½ h. Several additional focus groups were conducted in March and April 2009 to gain better insight into work/life issues as experienced by women in STEM. As a result of the feedback received, the program was retitled "Improving Work/Life Satisfaction", as the word "balance" did not effectively convey the complexity of the issues these professionals faced.

Concurrently, materials for the Program-In-A-Box toolkit for AWIS chapters were developed, including a facilitator's instruction guide, a workshop outline, a PowerPoint presentation, participant workbook, promotional material, participant self-evaluation instruments, and program evaluations. During the remainder of the year, on-site chapter programs contributed to further refinement of the workshop and accompanying materials.

In 2010, the program was presented to 14 additional AWIS chapters, reaching more than 340 individuals across the country. Outreach to scientific and professional societies was also initiated in 2010, with presentations at the Evolution 2010 Conference, the American Association of Medical Colleges Annual Meeting, and the University of New Mexico Mentoring Conference, reaching an additional combined total of approximately 250 people. As AWIS entered the third year of program development, continued outreach was accomplished via AWIS chapters across the United States in combination with targeted outreach to various professional scientific societies. The combined number of individuals who benefited from attending the Work/Life Satisfaction workshops in its first three years was more than 2500.

To sustain the program after the third year, the decision was made to bring in chapter leaders from around the country for a "Train the Trainer" session. Thirty chapter leaders were convened in 2011 for a 2-day Work/Life Satisfaction session during the AAAS Annual Meeting in Washington, DC. During this training, chapter leaders received professional development and program branding guidance. Ongoing chapter training was offered through Web-based programs during the remainder of the year. During these sessions, participants shared lessons learned and best practices and had their questions answered. Approximately 750 individuals have participated in the training program through the AWIS chapters and the Web-based programs through 2012.

To maximize exposure for the program, a number of scientific conferences and meetings were targeted. Between 2009 and mid-2013, the workshop was given more than 40 times at conventions, including the Advancement of Women in STEM Leadership Summit at Pfizer, Inc., the National Symposium for the Advancement of Women in Science at Harvard University, the Experimental Biology 2011 Conference, the Cambridge Science Festival, a meeting at Genentech, the annual meetings of the National Postdoctoral Association, the Society of Women Engineers, the Materials Research Society, and the American Geophysical Union, as well as the Joint Mathematics Meeting and the National Science Foundation's ADVANCE Program Meeting. The program was also presented at a number of universities including the University of Maryland, University of New Mexico, the Medical University of South Carolina, West Virginia University, University of Texas Southwestern Medical Center, Argonne National Laboratory, Louisiana Tech University, Iowa State University, University of California Davis, University of Delaware, Middle Tennessee State University, Drexel University, New Jersey Institute of Technology, Ohio State University, and Towson State University. As a result of this continuous and ongoing outreach, the program has reached directly more than 3000 individuals comprising men and women from a broad range of STEM disciplines.

Implementation Highlights

In the original survey and needs assessment, one of the questions asked for recommendations on the type of work/life programs that would best meet the respondents' needs. The responses included design and structure the work/life satisfaction resources for different ages and stages; establish networks and peer networking; and offer in-person, chapter-based local sessions. Due to the time pressures they faced, respondents also suggested that various types of resources be offered multiple times and in multiple formats.

To best meet this request, a focused effort was made to reach out to all AWIS chapters, either in person or by bringing the chapter leaders together for training. The aforementioned scientific conferences and other meetings of interest were selected, at which the program could be presented as a workshop, a panel session, or part of the poster presentation. In addition, a number of resources were made available to AWIS chapters and members:

- A Program-In-A-Box toolkit to help AWIS chapters launch their own work/life satisfaction programs at the local level. (All materials included in this toolkit are available to members on the AWIS Web site.) The kit's PowerPoint presentation is available in a number of versions to best meet the needs of the audience using it, as well as to best fit the time constraints that may exist in presenting this program at the local level.
- A workbook containing exercises for self-reflection and ongoing assessment based on what was learned during the on-site program. A resource guide providing suggested readings and links to Web sites focusing on the topic of work/life satisfaction was also included. The workbook and resource guide are also available on the AWIS Web site.

- Webinars to support ongoing learning for participants in local programs and beyond. These presentations did not supplant the "live" program offered through the local AWIS chapters but rather supplemented it. Each of the webinars focused on one component of the program (e.g., cultivating a strong support system through effective mentoring) to provide greater interaction and more in-depth discussion among the participants during the webinar itself.

Overall, the impact of the Improving Work/Life Satisfaction program has been significant. The program has been very well received by participants in a number of settings; modifications, based on both continuous assessment and evaluations by the participants, continue to be made along the way. The program has proven to be very adaptable to audience needs. A significant strength of the program is that it is very interactive, thus encouraging participants to share their stories and to learn from each other during and after the presentation.

Lessons Learned

Based on the participant evaluations, the number-one benefit of the program was the ability to interact with other attendees on a face-to-face basis. Even though 50% of the survey responses indicated that a face-to-face program was not critical, the informal networking component would have been completely lost in a "virtual" environment that did not include pre- and postworkshop interactions as participants entered and left the physical site. Individuals came away with a better understanding of the various issues that they needed to address as well as realizing that there were other people who were facing the same challenges they were and with whom they could interact later on for support and guidance. Many participants also noted that they felt alone in their struggles and were gratified to learn that other individuals found themselves in the same situation. This feeling of isolation was apparent at the beginning of each program and highlighted in the survey results. In light of this, the presenters realized the importance of creating an environment where participants felt that their comments would be kept confidential.

The nature of the scientific enterprise can be very stressful and highly competitive. Women in STEM say they benefit from meeting periodically to discuss issues of importance to them. Such face-to-face meetings may help in retaining those women who are contemplating leaving science.

Another lesson relates to one of the program's initial goals: offering ongoing coaching support through group sessions specifically designed to expand participants' peer-support systems. AWIS members who participated in the on-site educational program were offered additional fee-based group coaching sessions to deepen their learning experience. However, the response rate to the offer of follow-up coaching was low. More women said they were interested in follow-up peer mentoring, either in person or virtually. Additional consideration is now being given to developing a peer-mentoring network that allows individuals to stay connected after the program concludes and to continue to network with each other. Women in STEM perceive the need to remain in touch with each other through mentoring programs that provide them with the opportunity to share their experiences and to learn from each other as a way to avoid feelings of isolation.

Although the original focus of the program was on female scientists, the program has since been opened to include men as well. The initial programs were attended exclusively by women but, over time, a number of younger men (and some older ones) began to attend as they realized that they were now facing the same issues that women have been facing for a number of years. This fact corresponds with the research showing that men are becoming more involved with family responsibilities. The program was also expanded beyond scientists to include engineers, technologists, and mathematicians, as many of these individuals are also facing challenges relating to work/life satisfaction. Finally, since the topic of work/life satisfaction is of importance to all individuals in STEM, the program has been modified to appeal to businesses, pharmaceutical firms, and scientific laboratories, although for the near future universities will continue to be the primary target workplace.

Sustainability

Long-term sustainability of the work/life satisfaction program is being accomplished, in part, through the activities of AWIS chapters. As a result of the training received by the chapter leaders, more than 20 chapters have presented the Work/Life Satisfaction program since mid-2011. As noted, the program has also been presented at more than a dozen universities. Its reputation is growing, as more and more universities come to understand the importance of professional development and of providing their faculty, staff, and students with the tools needed to become and remain successful in STEM fields. The national AWIS office now markets the program as a benefit to institutional members of AWIS and continues its outreach to universities and business.

The initial response from AWIS members to the original survey conducted in the United States was very informative about the barriers to achieving work/life satisfaction faced by women in STEM. The survey instrument is robust, and many questions have been adapted and used to further investigate issues facing individuals in the STEM field at the global level. In this way, AWIS is expanding upon the data collected from the first survey and utilizing the information gathered to work toward workplace transformation and systemic change.

Conclusions

Until sweeping changes are made in how science is conducted, along with changes in society's views of working men and women, the topic of work/life satisfaction will continue to be an urgent one. Cost-effective child care, dual-career employment, equal opportunities for advancement, and options to work part time or job share are all important considerations that must be addressed. To facilitate networking about work/life satisfaction on a global level and to remove the feeling of isolation often experienced by individuals in STEM, the development of a worldwide mentoring platform is needed. Research has shown that mentoring provides a much higher level of job satisfaction and retention for individuals in STEM.[9] Many women scientists are struggling to overcome antiquated ideas on the role of women in universities, corporations, and government agencies. Successful mentoring by senior-level women who can provide career advice based on their own experiences would benefit these struggling scientists. In so doing, such mentors would be able to "give back" to their profession by sharing their knowledge and expertise. AWIS continues to examine the feasibility of this undertaking before proceeding further.

CASE STUDY 2. CREATION AND IMPLEMENTATION OF A PROGRAM FOR PERSONAL AND PROFESSIONAL DEVELOPMENT OF WOMEN SCIENTISTS IN AN EMERGING DEMOCRACY

Implementing organization: Maternal and Childcare Union, Tbilisi, Georgia (2008 Elsevier Foundation New Scholars Grant Awardee).

Project leaders: Maia Butsashvili, MD, PhD; Marina Topuridze, MD, MS; George Kamkamidze, MD, PhD; Maia Kajaia, MD, MS; Ekaterine Kldiashvili, MS, PhD; Nino Lomia, MD, PhD; Tamar Butsashvili, MS; and Roena Sukhiashvili, MS.

Rationale and Goals

Scientific, technological, and medical knowledge are fundamental tools for addressing critical issues facing the developing countries today, such as weak political, economic, social, and health are structures that have resulted in poverty, hunger, and disease. Georgia, like other emerging democracies, has in recent years recognized the need for a larger science and technology workforce in general and a dramatic increase in women's full participation in it in particular. During the Soviet era, Georgia espoused gender equality. The government's official position was that women possess equal access to education and training, employment, promotions, and fair remuneration, and that they were to be given an equal opportunity to participate in social, political, and cultural activities. Such statements reflected only an outward appearance of equality; in reality, men occupied all the highest research and administrative positions in the sciences. As a result, the system did not provide real opportunities for women to become leaders in these fields.

In the current era, Georgia, like other modernized societies, is becoming actively involved in the promotion of democratic values in research. However, because of lack of experience, female researchers still have few opportunities to develop their careers in different fields of science. While women now constitute more than half of all participants in the country's scientific and academic institutions, they remain underrepresented in leadership positions. One of the main factors underlying this discrepancy is women's obligation to prioritize the family, a value intrinsic to Georgia's history and culture.

The Maternal and Childcare Union's program therefore focused on promoting the personal and professional development of women scientists in Georgia. Several objectives were set: (1) identify the barriers that prevent women scientists from advancing in their fields; (2) create and implement leadership development and educational programs for women working at scientific and academic institutions; (3) create opportunities for the advancement of women in science and in the community at large; (4) create a Web site offering course materials and promoting peer mentoring; (5) promote opportunities to help women balance work, family, and lifestyle; (6) help women to establish interinstitutional, personal, and peer-mentoring networks to share strategies for pursuing scientific career advancement while balancing family obligations; and (7) provide women scientists who are members of minority groups in Georgia (Armenian, Azerbaijani, Russian, Ossetian, and Kurd) with the opportunity to network and develop the skills necessary to advance in their careers.

Project Description and Outcomes

Prior to commencing the project, the organization conducted a self-administered survey of groups of women working at various academic and medical institutions to assess their career satisfaction; characterize the environment at their institution in terms of ability to balance work and family, child-care and elder-care benefits, and gender balance; and to identify the perceived means of improvement and the need for educational intervention. The survey results were enlightening. Forty-one percent of respondents believed that they did not have the appropriate environment to maintain the balance between family and work. Only 49% considered conditions adequate at their institution to ensure that child care was available for women with children. While the vast majority of respondents did not indicate any gender-related problems at time of entry into a new job, 44% of participants stated that they did not have the appropriate environment to fully utilize their skills and knowledge. About half of the women said their motivation for working was for both professional interest and for income. The remainder stated that they worked either just for money or just for professional interest. Eleven percent noted that they did not have a job directly related to their education and background.

Interestingly, more women said they were able and willing to express new ideas and take initiatives within the family than they could do so in the workplace. At work, they perceive initiative to be men's prerogative. More than a third of the women surveyed (36%) thought that men's ideas were considered to be more important than those of women at their institution. For 44% of respondents, professional obligations caused disagreement within the family at some point, with 9% noting that this happened often. Women younger than 35 years were nine times more likely to consider their career advancement a priority in life compared with their older colleagues, for whom family obligations took a backseat to their scientific and career interests. Only 4% of the women surveyed had more than two children; only one participant had as many as four.

To begin to address some of the core issues revealed in the survey, a training framework was developed by specialists who had the appropriate knowledge and experience in each topic. Training courses, which included lectures and group discussions, were conducted in Georgia's capital, Tbilisi, for 153 project participants—women scientists at the doctoral level who were employed in medical and biological fields at the early career stages. Representatives of institutions in Tbilisi, as well as in other regions of the country, were enrolled in the project based on predefined selection criteria. Subgroups of women with similar backgrounds and interests were identified, with tailored training sessions conducted by the same group of specialists who developed the curriculum. Ten separate 1-week training courses were held, each consisting of a group of 15 women working in similar research areas. Most leaders of these training modules were themselves role models of women successful in their careers who were also exemplars of maintaining optimal balance between work and family obligations. The main topics covered during the 1-week training were promoting gender equality and empowering women in science and medicine; institutional change to promote gender equity; work and family balance; conflict-resolution skills; career planning and development; writing resumes and curriculum vitae and preparing for successful interviews; searching literature and writing research proposals; research ethics; preparing and publishing manuscripts; organizing and conducting interactive seminars and conferences; and creating and working with research tools such as databases.

As the project concluded, a final meeting of participating women was held. There they shared numerous success stories that demonstrated the program's efficacy in fostering a supportive network for women in Georgia. A presentation of the project's achievements was then made to representatives of academic and research institutions, the media, and policy makers. Attendance by a senior member of the Georgian Parliament resulted in subsequent coverage of her participation on a leading television channel in Georgia.

Implementation Highlights

Convening training sessions composed of women with similar professional interests and backgrounds was critical to the success of the project. The careful planning of the program topics and selection of participants enabled a more intensive interaction among the participants in each of the 10 sessions. In parallel with those on-site training programs in Tbilisi, a Web site was developed on which the lecture materials were posted, allowing free access by all interested individuals and by institutions that wished to use them for educational purposes. Three online seminars were also conducted during the course of the project. During the seminars, small groups of women and training-course leaders discussed their progress and challenges as well as project participants' questions. These seminars were originally intended as continuing activities after the 1-week training program. However, major impediments to efficiency and to significant expansion and utilization of the online seminars existed due to the limitations of Internet communication within Georgia. Not all women have access to personal computers and Internet access outside the capital. Hence, several participants encountered difficulties with online seminar participation. Also, while e-mail communication can be effective, a significant strength of the program lay in opportunities for direct interaction through verbal discussions. The challenges presented by technology limitations required significant adjustments during the course of implementation and follow-through. Nevertheless, creating an opportunity for women to establish connections with colleagues as a basis for future networking and potential research collaborations remained a central focus of the project.

Lessons Learned

It is very important to equip women from different regions and at different institutions in present-day Georgia with the tools, skills, and networks needed to advance their careers, balance family and work, and assume leadership positions. Strengthening specific academic skills, such as asking relevant research questions, developing competitive grant proposals, effectively managing research projects, and publishing results in peer-reviewed journals can have a significant positive impact on the advancement of women's careers in this nation.

The presentation of program results and achievements to the mass media, the academic and research communities, government ministries, and other policy makers was a very important step for the project. This wide exposure demonstrated the importance of empowering women scientists to advance their careers and the significance of such empowerment for the country at large. Another very important step was the development of recommendations, based on survey data and other information, to guide institutions in maximizing the potential of women in science and engineering careers in Georgia. These recommendations may now be used by faculty, deans, department chairs, and other university leaders; scientific and professional societies; funding organizations; and government agencies.

Sustainability

A document with recommendations developed during the project's final workshop was distributed to institutions across different sectors to help them improve recruitment and retention of women scientists and engineers in various positions. Project course materials and final recommendations were also placed on the central Web site.[10] All interested institutions are now able to use the educational course for their staff, and women enrolled in the program are sustaining their communication and peer-mentoring networks. Some of the participants have replicated the project for women at their own institutions.

Conclusions

The program was very effective, as most of the participants used the skills gained during the training course to move forward in their career development. Several success stories emerged of participating women scientists who developed curriculum vitae, applied for research scientist positions, had successful interviews, and became involved in the projects in which they were interested. Also, the program encouraged some of the participating women to continue working in their PhD programs concurrent with their family responsibilities (they were married and had children). Training in grant writing during the program helped numerous participants to develop research proposals and submit them to funding agencies, resulting in successful funding of scientific projects. It is anticipated that participants will continue to disseminate the program at their institutions and among their growing professional networks.

CASE STUDY 3. A WRITING RETREAT FOR WOMEN IN SCIENCE AND ENGINEERING

Implementing organization: University of Nebraska-Lincoln, Lincoln, Nebraska, USA (2011 Elsevier Foundation New Scholars Grant Awardee).

Project leaders: Patricia Wonch Hill, PhD; Mary Anne Holmes, PhD; and Julia McQuillan, PhD.

Rationale and Goals

A critical component of success in the STEM fields is the ability to convey the outcomes of one's research in writing and to prepare cogent proposals for funding one's research endeavors. The focus of this particular undertaking was to retain women in STEM fields by improving their writing and promoting social connections through networking. A multidisciplinary, multirank, weeklong writing retreat was envisioned. Unlike writers in STEM fields, those in the arts and humanities have long recognized the importance of using retreats to foster consistent writing and greater confidence in one's chosen profession. Hence, the retreat was intended to test this concept, offering coaching on professional writing, peer feedback, blocks of unstructured writing time to improve writing success, and group meals and accommodations to facilitate social connections among faculty participants. Specific goals were to (1) increase the number of publications by STEM women who attended the writing retreat and/or who participated in a subsequent interactive videoconference; (2) provide expert writing advice and coaching to enhance writing productivity and thereby lay a foundation for long-term writing success and higher professional productivity; and (3) assist participants in creating and facilitating social connections to share implicit knowledge about successful academic careers.

Project Description and Outcomes

The University of Nebraska-Lincoln (UNL) recently joined the Committee on Institutional Cooperation (CIC, "Big Ten"), which facilitates collaborative research through shared library resources and regular meetings among deans, department chairs, and heads of member institutions (the universities of Nebraska-Lincoln, Michigan, Wisconsin, Illinois, Maryland, Minnesota, Iowa, Chicago, Michigan State, and Indiana, plus Purdue, Ohio State, Rutgers, Northwestern, and Penn State universities). Building on current ties among the CIC institutions, the project sought to enrich those existing connections.[11] Three previous UNL-exclusive writing retreats and a writing retreat for women in the geosciences in the northeast United States provided background information on structure and content in creating a framework for this multi-institutional project.[12-14]

Such writing retreats provide an opportunity for junior and senior faculty to share disciplinary expertise, and this mutual exchange can enhance the professional confidence and knowledge of the women involved. In addition, participants can share insights on successfully managing time and work/life balance. The "Big Ten" STEM writing retreat built on and extended this framework, bringing together an existing network of institutions, multiple disciplines, and multiple ranks; offering facilitated, ongoing quarterly writing "accountability and support" videoconferences; and providing dependent-care support during the retreat. Because broad participation in the retreat was crucial, STEM women throughout UNL were invited to attend and asked to invite their collaborators and women with whom they would like to collaborate from other CIC institutions. Women STEM faculty members from across CIC institutions were also invited to participate.

In addition, the Bureau of Sociological Research at UNL conducted an experimental evaluation with participants to assess whether extended professional writing guidance, in the form of quarterly videoconferences after the retreat was over, could help women better achieve their writing goals. Such evaluation results were intended to determine the most cost-effective measures for supporting writing and academic success for women in STEM. Specific assessments were conducted to address success in reaching the project's stated goals as well as to compare outcomes in writing habits, publications, and networking among participants in both the retreat and videoconference, participants in the retreat only, and their departmental peers who did not participate in either the retreat or the videoconference.

Implementation Highlights

The retreat was advertised by writing directly to UNL women STEM faculty and by asking deans to ask department chairs to encourage their faculty to participate. Similar requests were made at five other CIC institutions (those with ADVANCE-IT grants). In addition, all UNL faculty members who registered were asked to nominate women faculty in STEM at CIC institutions whom they would like to meet and/or with whom they would like to work or were already working, to invite to the writing retreat. Twenty-one faculty members from five CIC institutions (including UNL) and five additional institutions ultimately attended. Faculty participants were from all ranks and included a broad range of STEM fields (anthropology, medicine, zoology, chemistry and biochemistry, statistics, environmental science, chemical and biomolecular engineering, civil engineering, geography, sociology, limnology, biology, and earth and atmospheric sciences). Two men attended: one as part of a dual-career couple and the other as the parent of young children.

Content was tailored to improving the quality and quantity of publications for STEM scientists. Because writing retreats traditionally have been geared toward the humanities, aspects of this retreat were modified to benefit writers in STEM fields. Critical postretreat aspects were the anticipated follow-up quarterly videoconferences and outcome surveys. Based on participant preference, four videoconferences were offered, providing information on publishing, the tenure process, leadership, and issues related to increasing retention of women in STEM fields in academia.

To prepare for the writing retreat, held in June 2012, selected faculty were asked to describe their writing goals for the retreat and to complete a short pretest survey to provide baseline data about themselves. Because a major barrier for women STEM faculty is balancing work and family life, accommodating the greater caregiving needs of women scientists was a prominent feature of the writing retreat. Participants were encouraged to bring their school-aged children to the retreat, where the children would attend a weeklong STEM-related summer day camp provided by the Lincoln Children's Museum. Children too young to attend camp were accommodated on an individual basis, depending on age and needs of the participant. Participants who were parents of young children were also eligible for a stipend to help cover the costs of caregiving while they were attending the retreat. Twelve children attended overall, with a broad age range spanning from 2 months to 9 years.

Lessons Learned

The schedule and format of the retreat were key to its ultimate success. Structured mealtimes were expected to be used for informal networking. With faculty participants arriving on a Sunday night, an initial "icebreaker" event was held at which participants shared their goals for the retreat. Monday was designated as unstructured writing time for all participants. On Tuesday, a faculty member whose expertise is in science writing led a half-day writing workshop on writing effectively in the sciences. This session was followed by scheduled meetings for individualized feedback. Because participants were encouraged to send a copy of their projects to the writing coach ahead of time, more in-depth review and feedback could occur in those sessions. Wednesday and Thursday offered more unstructured writing time, with a presentation held on Thursday afternoon on STEM women in academia. One of the unexpected benefits of the writing retreat was the camaraderie forged between the scientist-parents. Participants were able to both discuss work/family integration and see it in practice.[15,16]

Sustainability

After the retreat, all participants were mailed the same short outcome survey at 6 and 12 months to assess their progress toward establishing writing habits, reaching individual goals, and establishing formal and informal social networking. The aforementioned three-group experimental design will serve to inform assessment of outcomes. Group A attended the retreat and had the option to take part in a facilitated follow-up and a quarterly 1-h videoconference. Group B attended the retreat and received only the 6- and 12-month outcome surveys. Group C comprised the control group, peers in the participants' departments. They received only a 5-min Web survey at 12 months postretreat. This group will be used for comparison of writing habits and publication outcomes with the two participant groups. By mid-2014, the project team members plan to create a short guide to facilitating STEM writing retreats and to publish a study outlining the different types of writing retreats available to STEM and non-STEM academics, along with an overview of the results from evaluation of this particular writing retreat. Initial outcomes were encouraging: the 6 months postretreat survey showed great success in terms of participants' productivity. Among the 17 people who completed the pre- and postretreat surveys, seven papers have been submitted and two of those have been published. In addition, two books and a book chapter have been submitted for publication. Finally, four participants wrote grants; two were not awarded, but two have been funded.

Conclusions

The ongoing quarterly online webinars are aimed at maintaining the social ties and leveraging the momentum created at the writing retreat. Participants are invited for a 1-h phone call with experts in science writing. At the time of the 6-month postretreat survey, four respondents reported keeping in contact with people they met at the writing retreat. An unanticipated result of the retreat was that many participants went back to their home institutions and created their own writing groups. Two writing groups as well as two mini retreats were formed by participants. In addition, many participants reported that they have better writing habits since attending the retreats and webinars. Another promising preliminary finding was that individuals who attended the retreat were statistically significantly more likely to report that they have "a writing schedule that is inviolate" ($p < 0.05$).

PRACTICAL TOOLS

Core Questions and Concepts to Guide Participants in Examining Their Approaches to Work/Life Satisfaction

(Adapted from the AWIS Improving Work/Life Satisfaction program materials and workshops.)

What is your biggest work/life challenge?

Who/what do you use for a support system?

Who/what could you add to your support system?

Think of something you have been asked to do recently, and then ask yourself these five questions:

1. Must this be done?
2. Must this be done by me?
3. Must this be done right now?
4. Must this be done this way?
5. If I say yes to this, what am I saying no to?

Also: Is there a way that you can say NO by saying YES ("Here is what I *CAN* do")?

Think of a situation that causes you a lot of stress or anxiety. How can you shift your mind-set to make yourself mentally prepared/tough enough to deal with it?

Think of one thing that makes you feel guilty. What boundaries can you establish to remain guilt free?

Think of one thing that you could ask for that would help you with your work/life satisfaction.

What are the top five things that you need to do in the next week for work? In your personal life?

What are three things that you will do this week to recharge your batteries?

Reflect back on your responses to the above questions and identify one change you would like to make that will improve your personal work/life satisfaction. Then consider the following.

One change that I can make in the next 30 days that will improve my personal work/life satisfaction is:

One benefit of making this change is:

Three roadblocks that could get in the way of making this change are:

My plan for overcoming these obstacles is:

The people I will ask to support me in making this change are:

I will track my progress toward making this change by:

For individual reflection:

Think about a current personal or professional choice that is out of alignment with your priorities and values.

What is the short- or long-term benefit of this choice?
Why is this important to me?
What is the cost of this choice? Is the cost worth it to me?
Is there another choice I could make that would increase my work/life satisfaction?

An Agenda for a Successful Writing Retreat

(Adapted from the University of Nebraska-Lincoln's 5-day writing retreat held June 17–22, 2012.)

A well thought-out agenda for writing retreats affirms that unstructured time is critical to the process. Useful approaches include welcoming and orientation sessions, a writing coach session, and social time to foster networking. In general, activities should be kept to a minimum and writing time to a maximum. UNL's first retreat schedule provides an example.

Sunday, June 17
2:00 p.m.–6:00 p.m.	Check-in at Kauffman Residential Center, UNL Campus
6:00 p.m.	Reception at the Nebraska State Museum; welcome and introductions

Monday, June 18
6:30 a.m.–8:30 a.m.	Breakfast at Selleck Dining Hall
8:00 a.m.	Attendees with special dining needs meet at Selleck
8:30 a.m.	Meet Children's Museum staff at Kauffman, optional visit to museum
8:30 a.m.–11:00 a.m.	Unstructured writing time
11:00 a.m.–1:00 p.m.	Lunch—Selleck Dining Hall
1:00 p.m.–4:30 p.m.	Unstructured writing time
4:30 p.m.	Children return from Children's Museum
5:00 p.m.–7:00 p.m.	Dinner—Selleck Dining Hall

Tuesday, June 19
6:30 a.m.–8:30 a.m.	Breakfast at Selleck Hall
8:30 a.m.	Meet Children's Museum staff at Kauffman
9:00 a.m.–11:00 a.m.	Writing coach presentation, Kauffman Room 110
11:00 a.m.–1:00 p.m.	Lunch—Selleck Dining Hall
1:00 p.m.–4:30 p.m.	Unstructured writing time
4:30 p.m.	Children return from Children's Museum
5:00 p.m.–7:00 p.m.	Dinner—Selleck Dining Hall
7:00 p.m. (optional)	Jazz in June, on the plaza west of the Sheldon Museum of Art

Wednesday, June 20
6:30 a.m.–8:30 a.m.	Breakfast at Selleck Hall
8:30 a.m.	Meet Children's Museum staff at Kauffman
8:30 a.m.–11:30 a.m.	Unstructured writing time
11:00 a.m.–1:00 p.m.	Lunch—Selleck Dining Hall
1:00 p.m.–4:30 p.m.	Unstructured writing time
5:00 p.m.–7:00 p.m.	Dinner—Selleck Dining Hall
4:30 p.m.	Children return from Children's Museum
	Ice cream social on the lawn

Thursday, June 21
6:30 a.m.–8:30 a.m.	Breakfast at Selleck Dining Hall
8:30 a.m.	Meet Children's Museum staff at Kauffman
8:30 a.m.–11:30 a.m.	Unstructured writing time
11:00 a.m.–1:00 p.m.	Lunch—Selleck Dining Hall
1:00 p.m.–4:30 p.m.	Unstructured writing time
4:30 p.m.	Children return from Children's Museum
5:00 p.m.–7:00 p.m.	Dinner—Selleck Dining Hall
6:00 p.m.–8:00 p.m.	Music at the Children's Museum
Friday, June 22	Departure day; breakfast and lunch available at Selleck

Dual Careers and Strategic Decision Making

Being unwilling to move cities because I was happy with my children's school adversely affected my career. —**A male scientist, age 56–65 years, married/ partnered, Switzerland**

Equitable Solutions for Retaining a Robust STEM Workforce.
http://dx.doi.org/10.1016/B978-0-12-800215-5.00004-X

Other than placing my spouse on my healthcare plan, my spouse does not exist in the eyes of the institution. **—A man working in arts and humanities, age 36–45 years, married/partnered, USA**

Taking control of one's scientific career is critical for professional success and for overall life satisfaction. This process begins with the complex decisions that must be made in the context of a scientist's professional development, career path, and "away from work" life. For many female scientists, the dual-career household presents ongoing dilemmas for themselves and their partners or spouses. Both individuals are most likely striving for meaningful, productive, and challenging professional work in accord with their interests and training. Even those for whom the dual-career dilemma is not relevant must make strategic and complex decisions about their professional pathway and how it intersects with their overall life interests. To date, there have been few obvious approaches that can be deployed to resolve these conflicts. As well, there has been very little study in the real-life laboratory of the workplace of how organizations and institutions can support individuals in their decision making about career and life options. This chapter presents two case studies of Elsevier New Scholars projects, each of which takes a significantly different approach to the dual-career issue and to the context of making strategic work/life decisions. Both address the dual-career dilemma and the strategic (and often difficult) choices that scientists must make.

Case study 4 describes an approach undertaken by a university that was experiencing difficulty in recruiting and retaining female science and engineering faculty. The project leaders noted that some turnover in career paths is demographically specific, occurring particularly among women who are pursuing significant work and family duties at the same time. Such women may choose to leave a company or institution instead of sacrificing their other interests and responsibilities in order to make the job work out. Other women elect to quit their jobs after giving birth rather than simply taking a maternity leave. Further, women's perceptions of their career paths might lower their level of commitment to any particular firm or institution because they believe they are not in contention for top-level jobs. These factors, along with spousal employment and postchildbirth (or adoption) family issues, can at many companies and institutions translate into higher voluntary turnover rates for women. This higher attrition is also costly to institutions, as professionals and top executives typically are the most expensive hires and at the most risk for turnover. Case study 4 presents a creative approach to dealing with these issues in which the evolution of the initial effort evolved into a successful nonprofit organizational model that could be widely adopted. It is a superb example of a strong university-community partnership.

Case study 5 describes the development of a new approach to enabling female scientists at the critical early stages of their careers to make more informed and more appropriate career decisions and plans. The project leaders were motivated by the need to address the issues that individuals face in balancing career aspirations and family responsibilities, child care issues and costs, mobility, dual careers, and returning after career breaks. Facilitating the individual's consideration of four key aspects of her career is a central focus. These aspects include the employing institution and job-specific issues; her expected research output and impact; engagement in and recognition by the scientific community; and personal beliefs, attitudes, and circumstances. This case study also presents a framework that institutions can deploy to help the individual female scientist understand and navigate the complex relationships between events and decisions that shape her professional development through the doctoral and postdoctoral stages.

CASE STUDY 4. DUAL-CAREER SOLUTIONS AND OTHER MEANINGFUL APPROACHES TO RECRUITMENT AND RETENTION EFFORTS

Implementing organization: Tech Valley Connect, created by Rensselaer Polytechnic Institute, Troy, New York, USA (2007 Elsevier Foundation New Scholars Grant Awardee).

Project leaders: Cheryl Geisler, PhD; Robert Palazzo, PhD; Deborah Kaminski, PhD; and Angela McNerney, Program Director (now President and Executive Director).

Rationale and Goals

Tech Valley Connect (TVC) (then called PhD Move) began as a pilot program in 2009 to address dual-career challenges for women in science. The initiative focused on retention of newly relocating faculty, providing unique settling-in services to help transition the new hire's family to their new environment. The original program focused on this approach because research had shown that both spousal employment and family assimilation issues were top reasons that new hires were lost within the first 3 years.[17–19] This loss of retention is costly—conservative estimates show two to three times the salary of the original hire.[20,21] The program was developed as the result of a number of investigations the group undertook to identify core issues and to envision solutions.

The process began with a series of interviews with women on the Rensselaer Polytechnic Institute (RPI) faculty who experienced an unsupported settling-in process with an accompanying partner.[22] Based on this information and discussions with various industry sector employers, the group developed a prototype plan for addressing retention that focused on developing comprehensive and innovative services to meet the need for spousal employment by reaching beyond the bounds of the university and gaining commitment from regional businesses across various industries. After these initial concepts were developed and the model further refined, a nonprofit organization was created that now provides unique economic development infrastructure in the Capital Region of New York.[23]

Project Description and Outcomes

TVC is an innovative nonprofit organization composed of a consortium of capital region employers focused on recruitment and retention of professionals. Trailing spouse/accompanying partner issues are a major worry for both the employer who is concerned with retention and for many candidates who are considering placement in a new location. TVC provides detailed services to newly relocated professionals and their families, helping them with spousal employment, family assimilation, and cultural transitions. The program has become a strong part of upstate New York's regional infrastructure, helping to bolster local economies while significantly increasing retention rates for area employers.

The program is activated when members of the consortium (employers) refer new hires and their families to a TVC family coordinator. Once the coordinator has made contact, an in-depth evaluation session is scheduled at which the family can speak confidentially with this individual, who will be assigned to them for 1 year. The spouse/partner employment-assistance model is unique in that coordinators arrange networking opportunities with decision makers from within the consortium in the spouse/partner's discipline. These informational interviews are not for specific openings but rather an opportunity to gain access to management in one's field and begin the process of building a substantial professional network. Face-to-face meetings have a more powerful impact on the employment search than looking at job postings and e-mailing resumes. The conversation is more specific than at a formal interview and the dynamics of the meeting change because the discussion is informal. Spouses/partners gain an opportunity to meet professionals who may have inside knowledge of opportunities in the field, such as colleagues who are seeking quality candidates. Or, they may know of others in their field to whom they can introduce the spouse/partner, broadening his or her web of contacts. This approach is consistent with the National Bureau of Labor Statistics finding that more than 70% of all employed individuals found their jobs through some form of networking. In the professions, this rate is most likely higher, as these populations are the riskiest in terms of retention.

The TVC family coordinator addresses assimilation first by conducting a thorough, six-page evaluation of the family to determine their needs and the specific resources available to them. A customized portfolio is prepared for each family, connecting them to qualified, vetted resources within the capital region. In this way, TVC coordinators become a confidential sounding board for the family, steering them toward resources that will ultimately create a better quality of life.

Because foreign nationals face even greater challenges when relocating, in 2012, TVC launched its Cultural Transition Program to help assimilate people to the culture, customs, and traditions of the United States. Partnerships with area groups associated with the international sector were forged to create well-rounded educational workshops. The workshops cover a comprehensive agenda, including topics such as education, health care, banking, government, and households. It is anticipated that the Cultural Transition Program will become central to the region as efforts to accommodate a more sophisticated international population increase. Here again, focused guidance to local resources is a strong point, allowing families to acquire the tools they need for a successful transition. In addition, staff members involved with the program have been certified in Cross Cultural Competence by the Interchange Institute in Boston, Massachusetts.

Another program created by TVC to help professionals integrate into the capital region is the Strategic Volunteer Initiative. This effort consists of a structured community service program connecting newly relocated professionals with volunteer opportunities in the region. Volunteering in a community facilitates professional and personal networking and hence, builds the relationships needed to strengthen ties to the area. About 20% of the families availing themselves of TVC services are foreign nationals whose spouse/partner may not have a work visa. TVC connects them to a nonprofit organization whose mission is closely connected to the spouse's professional background and where he or she can volunteer services. Such activities help keep the individuals professionally relevant as well as offsetting resume gaps. The time commitment for volunteering serves as both a means to meet people who share common interests and those closely affiliated with their own profession. In this way, it allows the spouse/partner to become integrated into the region both socially and professionally.

TVC's metric for success has been retention of the original hire. According to surveys conducted by the National Bureau of Labor Statistics, the average national voluntary turnover rate in 2012 was 9.8% and climbing. This number may be significantly higher when targeting professionals. TVC, as an independent nonprofit programme for more than 3 years, is operating below its target of 4.7% voluntary turnover with the riskiest population. By reducing turnover by roughly 50%, the program has been able to keep significant dollars not only within the region, but also within the employer-member organizations themselves. If this significant drop in voluntary turnover continues, TVC considers that it will have made significant strides in addressing the dual-career issue.

Because TVC addresses spousal employment and family assimilation issues directly by offering appropriate services, it is expected that the regional retention rate will increase for the employers within the consortium. In addition, because TVC is the first and so far only organization in the country with a demonstrated commitment from regional employers to spousal employment, it is helping to further distinguish the capital region from competing regions in terms of attracting new businesses and talent. As of July 2013, the consortium membership has grown from 12 institutions in the pilot phase to 63 institutions.

Implementation Highlights

The pilot program, which ran from July 2009 to December 2009, brought together 12 large employers crossing industry sectors to form a consortium committed to providing informational interviews for spouse/ partners of new hires at RPI. This pilot phase demonstrated that each identified industry faced similar retention challenges and was eager for meaningful solutions.

A TVC family coordinator (see above) was hired to work with new employees and their families; this individual would be referred to them by consortium members (employers). The pilot program provided insights into retention and dual-career issues. However, in order to measure retention accurately, at least five additional years will be required to demonstrate that the metric has been successfully met.

After conclusion of the 6-month pilot program, an analysis found sufficient positive feedback from participants, and unanimous agreement among the consortium members, to justify continuing the program as a nonprofit 501(c)(3) organization. In January 2010, a strong Board of Directors was established, along with an Advisory Board. These boards provide invaluable expertise, and the diversity among employer-members has created the equivalent of a powerful think tank to support the program. Although a basic Web site was designed and launched soon after the pilot began, later a need was seen for a more effective online presence. After the program's transition to nonprofit status, sponsorship was enlisted for development of a more user-friendly Web site.

The project has been well publicized, both regionally and nationally. Marketing materials have been developed and used to engage new organizations and bring them into the consortium. Monthly social events were also initiated to engage consortium members in social and professional networking. As more organizations and local businesses became TVC "sponsors", others desiring exposure to newly relocated professionals and their families soon followed suit. A quarterly newsletter has kept clients engaged, as have weekly e-mail "blasts" announcing local events and interesting venues. The newsletter also spotlights consortium members, profiles dual-career clients, and keeps employers and the business community at large apprised of current information and statistics regarding relocating employees.

Lessons Learned

TVC, like any start-up, has grown and faced challenges over the first years of its existence. During the pilot phase, many important conclusions were reached and resulted in a change of direction that helped the entity mature into an organization not originally envisioned. The following aspects now define the program:

- Initially, TVC's goals were to offer spouses/partners three informational interviews and a check-in with families/clients each quarter. The pilot experience revealed that job seekers needed many more than three professional contacts and that engagement was needed on a more regular basis. TVC now checks in with clients once a month after the initial contact is made and invites these families to monthly social events where they can meet other professionals and newly relocated people facing similar challenges.
- It was vital that TVC become an independent organization to maintain neutral relationships with all the consortium members, as many are competing institutions. The current model works within its status as an independent nonprofit entity funded by consortium membership fees, sponsorship grants, and donated resources.
- TVC expanded its scope to include all professionals (not just holders of PhD degrees) as its target clients. Such inclusiveness creates a stronger basis for involvement by many more companies, organizations, and institutions. Dual-career issues do not discriminate, and this issue affects most industries.
- The interactive Web site initially planned proved to be expensive and difficult to implement and manage. Work with a Web site designer led instead to the design of an efficient and informative site where clients could find answers quickly.
- Because TVC's clients belonged to a high-end professional demographic, businesses in the capital region eagerly sought exposure to them. This knowledge was extremely useful in obtaining vetted sponsors to help support the program.
- As the model grows, TVC is looking to build stronger partnerships and to gain momentum in tapping the market in the capital region in order to stimulate better cash flow and ensure the program's

sustainability. Getting all partners to engage fully has been a slow process, because they themselves are still testing whether this model will be a successful one for them. Many first sign up to be an Associate Member, a status that provides them an opportunity to conduct informational interviews and attend social events. The next step is for them to refer their new hires to TVC. However, arranging introductions to an employer's leadership can sometimes be difficult. Not all employers maintain open connections between human resources personnel and those in top positions. Buy-in from the highest levels at employer organizations is essential for the informational interview portion of the program to be effective.

- Because economic environments can change, it is important for expectations to remain flexible, as well as to obtain commitments in writing.
- The quality of TVC's Board of Directors had made a dramatic difference in the success of the program because the board has been able to engage key leaders in the community across many disciplines.

Sustainability

The next goal is challenging—to disseminate the TVC model to the entire capital region and surrounding communities. For this to happen, it will be necessary to increase the marketing budget substantially and, at the very least, double partnerships. Currently, services are marketed through word of mouth, limited marketing materials, the Web site, and the continued efforts of staff. With new memberships, the program would grow, thus adding to the critical mass necessary to produce results that would be meaningful on a national level.

Fortunately, in 2012, implementation of the Cultural Transition program provided TVC with another revenue stream. Workshops were developed for teaching United States culture to newly relocated foreign nationals and diversity-training seminars were offered to employees of consortium members, preparing them to work with international clientele and global businesses. The workshops cover municipalities and government, civil rights and laws, household differences, and banking and credit histories, along with United States history, culture, customs, traditions, and health care and education systems. The seminars included detailed information regarding doing business with specific nationalities and covered topics such as relationships and respect, communication, initial contacts and meetings, negotiation, decision making, agreements and contracts, and women in business.

Recently, TVC was contacted by five universities that requested consulting services to help them replicate the model. Three of these requests were in response to a supplemental grant offered by the National Science Foundation ADVANCE programs for initiatives addressing career/life balance. As of mid-August 2013, one of the universities had indicated they had received grant funding and TVC has begun working with this institution. TVC intends to continue to provide comprehensive consulting services to help replicate the program across the country.

Conclusion

This program model has been tested in a community with large employers from varying sectors and found to be highly effective. TVC's clients are staying in their jobs. In the brief period since the program's initial implementation, TVC has worked with 114 clients and their families, and has lost only five original hires.

This success demonstrates that the extraordinary cost of losing an employee shortly after they have relocated can be mitigated with the intervention provided by this model, and that the employers are willing to pay for a means of increasing retention. The personalized and individualized support for the family of a new hire can be very effective in ensuring the entire family becomes settled into their new community. Moreover, the tangible resources offered by TVC can make the scale tip in the region's favor when business leaders consider moving their organizations to the capital region. In addition, when heavily recruited talent considers whether the spouse/partner will have meaningful opportunities for employment if a new position is accepted, these individuals may rest assured that they will have access to a structured organization that attends to their specific needs over the course of 1 year.

Having an organization in place that meets some of the dual-career needs of professionals, particularly one with a structured commitment to spousal employment in the region, can help build a solid infrastructure for relocating professionals, especially women. Attracting new businesses to the community is also a potential and desired outcome of the program.

CASE STUDY 5. A SCENARIO TOOLKIT FOR ADVANCING CAREERS IN SCIENCE

Implementing organization: Portia Ltd, London, England (2011 Elsevier Foundation New Scholars Grant Awardee).

Project leaders: Elizabeth Pollitzer, PhD; Martina Schraudner, PhD; and Adina Breiman, PhD.

Rationale and Goals

Portia Ltd, a nonprofit organization based in the United Kingdom, designs and implements effective strategies for gender equality in the fields of science, engineering, and technology. For this particular project, the organization developed a method to plan and run workshops designed with experts on the Scenario Method and tested at science institutions with relevant target participants. The Scenario Method provides participants with a framework in which they insert their own values, interests, and priorities as they reflect upon a number of alternative hypothetical futures for themselves. The creation of guidelines and materials—a "toolkit"—for different categories of participants was a key aspect of the approach. Such target groups included researchers, research supervisors, human resources departments, and research and promotion committees within institutions. Another key aspect was the creation of online resources containing information to assist participants during preparation for, or as part of, scenario building around career choices and decisions (e.g., facts about implicit gender bias in assessment and selection, workplace policies, harassment, mobility schemes, and research funding programs). The overall goal of the project was to adapt the participatory method of scenario construction for use as a tool to enable science institutions to support their researchers, in particular women at early career stages, in making more informed and effective professional- and personal-development decisions about career-related issues.[24]

Project Description and Outcomes

The motivation for this project arose from Portia Ltd's wide variety of accumulated experience related to and investigations of women's careers in science. Some of the persistent issues that influence women's careers were central to the conceptual framework used. These issues included the tendency of women's research interests to cluster in the life sciences; participation in networks that is less extensive than men's[25]; reluctance to apply for promotion even when ready[26]; ensuring a smooth return to the workforce after a career break such as returning to school to earn a PhD or taking a first postdoctoral position[27]; work/life balance, in that social institutions lag behind advances in employment[28]; dual-career couples and the "trailing spouse"[29]; significant gender differences in attitudes toward intellectual risk taking[30]; research publication rates as affected by personal and employment factors[31]; lower grant-application rates for women[32]; and bias in assessment, with assumptions of sameness and/or equity between women and men when there are genuine differences.[33] These and other issues and findings[34,35] served to inform the approach.

A scientist's career is more than a sequence of jobs or work roles. Traditional jobs and work are situated within and defined by the work organization, and are conducted for the benefit of that organization. This generalization may also apply to industry-based research and development positions, but in general, the scientist's main obligation is to help advance scientific knowledge. This commitment involves each individual in a variety of activities: interpreting the existing knowledge, identifying gaps in that knowledge, deriving new tasks for filling these gaps, conducting the tasks, and publishing new knowledge. The scientific community (and not, in general, the employing organization) is the arbiter of the relevance of the tasks undertaken and standards followed when research is conducted. The main role of the scientific institution that actually employs the scientist is to provide the necessary resources for this work, such as salary, equipment, and time to conduct research.

As noted, the novel aspect of this project concerns adapting the participatory method of scenario construction for use as a tool to assist science institutions in supporting their researchers—and in particular, women researchers at early career stages—by enabling these researchers to make more informed and effective professional- and personal-development decisions. Traditionally, the Scenario Method has been used in social policy settings to help direct attention to driving forces, possible avenues of change, and the span of contingencies that may be confronted when developing new ideas and plans. Here, the method was adapted to focus on events and decision points that influence the direction and progress of an individual's science career.

While many institutions have tried to address these issues through mentoring schemes, mostly in a one-on-one format, the dynamic and complex nature of scientific employment today means that a much wider range of experience and knowledge is needed to enable young researchers to explore all relevant career-related factors in their decision making. The group-based and participatory nature of the Scenario Method promotes sharing of knowledge and experience, peer learning, and team spirit and collaboration. Participants identify and analyze (1) available career choices and pathways (e.g., within the researcher's current institution, in their country, or abroad); (2) prevailing trends (e.g., globalization of research and development capacity and gender quotas); (3) events that may alter the environment in the future (e.g., new research funding, new maternity and employment laws); and (4) the roles of various categories of stakeholders (e.g., "gatekeepers", advisors, strategists, networks, and policy makers).

The exploratory framework thus allows construction of the science career in terms of three separate but interdependent components: *cognitive career, community career, and organizational career.*[36] The rationale for adapting the workshop concept to suit the Scenario Method is based on recent research showing that a scientist's career is composed of the three contexts named above: as a productive researcher, as a member of the science community, and as an employee of a science institution, respectively. The interplay among these contexts is shown in Figure 4.19, below. Structured in this way, career development becomes a task

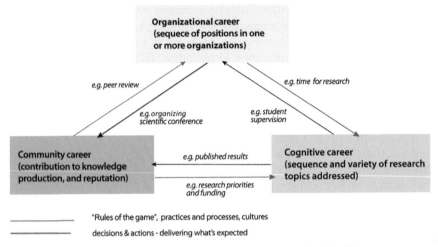

FIGURE 4.19 Three interdependent components of a scientific career.

of achieving a balance between these three areas of responsibility, plus any aspirations for a full private and family life. To do this effectively, an individual would need a much wider range of support measures than are possible through mentoring alone. For example, one of the key conditions for success in science is the ability to demonstrate intellectual independence (i.e., generate new and original research ideas). Another is the status granted to the individual by her scientific community (e.g., invitations to join important committees and boards or to serve as a keynote speaker at important conferences). These two key aspects shape the possible scenarios under which career pathways can be formed, depending on the scientist's ability to demonstrate intellectual independence, her professional ambition, and her professional and personal circumstances.

The motivation for producing a "Scenario Toolkit" was to help women, and in particular those in early career stages, to explore and virtually test possible career pathways by engaging in group-based activities involving a variety of individuals who can support the decision-making process. In this way, women will become more confident in the decisions they ultimately make about the direction and scope of their professional future. A critical phase in this process follows the completion of the PhD, when most researchers become intellectually independent from both the organization that employs them and their scientific community. At this point, they must make choices about research topics they want to address or methodologies they will explore. In fact, achieving such independence of thought is one of the key conditions that determine opportunities for advancement in a scientific career. This phase, then, is the most urgent one in terms of ensuring that the cognitive, organizational, and community careers are aligned. This intense consideration has to happen during the early career stage, a period when more women than men leave science.[37]

Implementation Highlights

In the early phases of the project, Portia Ltd formulated the scenario-building conditions, which included such factors as information on the process itself, micro- and macroelements influencing decisions, scenario logic(s), and decision strategies. The first priority was to establish the underlying logic to imagine a realistic future. In the context of scientific careers, *intellectual independence* and *professional status* are the two most valued measures of success, and hence offered two key dimensions for defining the scenario logic.

The four scenarios outlined in Figure 4.20 are as follows: scenario 1—lower independence and lower status (e.g., having a high teaching load, little time for research, and poor direction/support from colleagues, as well as a specialized research topic and facing many influential gate-keepers); scenario 2—high intellectual independence and lower status (e.g., having a self-selected but narrow research topic and sufficient time for research in a community that is small or with little influence in the "science system"); scenario 3—lower intellectual independence and higher status (e.g., having a research topic in a highly specialized field with work conducted in a renowned center of excellence with strong gatekeepers in a wide and influential community); and scenario 4—high intellectual independence and high status in the scientific community (e.g., having a research topic in a high-priority area and extensive collaborative networks in a community that influences key strategic/policy decisions).

An individual's career can shift from one scenario to another, and keen awareness of the different drivers that may influence these transitions can greatly help in the management of career progression. Awareness of factors that may influence career decision making is particularly important for women at early career stages. In scenario 1, for example, a researcher may have gained her PhD, continued with postdoctoral studies at the same institution, and been hired by the same institution later on. This may be a happy outcome in terms of stable employment and minimum disruption, but not one expected of a "top-level" scientist. In contrast, in scenario 4, another researcher may have moved between institutions, ensuring each time that the position she takes is in a top laboratory and involves top-level research groups. This person diligently produces publications, networks with top scientists, and takes initiative to be "visible" within her research community. To add a sense of reality to these scenarios, the project used a novel approach—the addition of role models—to demonstrate

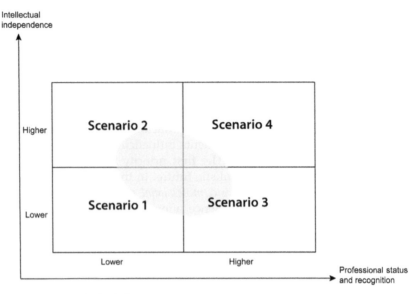

FIGURE 4.20 Scenarios of professional success.

the diversity of possible career paths both within and between the four scenarios. Invited experts in this process included representatives from human resources, research supervisors, research grant-awarding bodies, and other key actors in the research landscape. These experts facilitated an interactive engagement in the workshop with the participants, encouraging them to ask questions about their career choices, decisions, and ideas. Including role models as part of the Scenario Method facilitated the use of selected real-world examples that could be used for "back casting", a process in which individuals' career paths and decisions are traced from the present to an earlier starting point (in most cases, acquisition of the PhD).

Lessons Learned

In the first year of the project, the scenario approach was successfully adapted to create a workshop concept and design that can be implemented in different institutional settings and modified for local circumstances and resources. The adaptation of the Scenario Method for the purposes described above is new, and a new type of intervention is likely to emerge from its use. Both individuals and organizations will be able to use this methodology, which should also be easily adaptable across cultures, disciplines, and organizational settings. Although the work/life balance issue has been widely discussed, there continues to be a shortage of research studies on how female (and male) scientists construct the role of the family and other work/life issues in their career decision processes. Further understanding of this area would help individuals (and those mentoring them) to address this challenge more effectively. There is also a need to develop a good way to help women at early career stages to create a balanced perspective on dealing with the often conflicting societal forces they face. For example, there exists strong approval of women's pursuit of higher education, but equally strong approval of their full commitment to family life.

One way to help women scientists at early career stages to become more confident about their career aspirations when family pressures are the highest is to present them with a sufficient number of role models— different women who have established successful but varied career paths. Large and growing databases of women scientists provide a rich resource for discovering the potential diversity of career steps that are possible and how they may be combined into an effective career pathway. One example is Academia Net, which represents a database of 1200 women from primarily European countries.[38] Although the use of role models is often discussed in the context of women's participation in science, there is very little research evidence discussing their deployment in supporting career decision making.

Sustainability

Now that it has been developed, the Scenario Toolkit will be introduced through Portia's networks, which have grown over the last few years as a result of the organization's lead role in the European projects genSET and Gender Summit.[39,40] These networks will include EURODOC (an association for doctoral and postdoctoral researchers), the genSET Stakeholder Network (comprising more than 150 science institutions), and Portia's contact database of 45,000 people working in science in Europe and beyond. The pilot phase in year one demonstrated that the workshop designed around the Scenario Method could be translated into a practical and effective program that is adaptable to different institutional and national settings. The scenario approach has been shown to be successful in challenging participants to consider different possibilities and to think "outside the box", as well as enabling them to reach a balance between what they are capable of achieving, what they aspire to, and what they must do in order to establish a career path that is best for them in their current circumstances. The final product will be created after an evaluation workshop in 2014 that will bring together target users of the Scenario Method Toolkit (institutions, associations, and employers).

Conclusions

It is anticipated that the toolkit will enhance the capacity of young female scientists to make career decisions that are the best for them by exploring key concepts including understanding the available career options; gaining perspectives on how the "system" works; recognizing and choosing the right role models; avoiding cultural stereotypes; and addressing family-life issues. The scenario-based approach goes beyond traditional mentorship by providing an innovative strategy to better support female scientists and engineers in career development. Significantly, the concept not only works for female junior researchers, but also appeals to a male audience. Its value for institutions lies in their ability to use the workshops to help female scientists navigate the complex relationships between events and decisions that shape a professional career through the doctoral and postdoctoral stages. The concept comes at a timely moment, as institutions debate the best ways to facilitate workforce development and deployment. The program's holistic, scenario-based approach offers a way for institutions to support individuals in successfully making more informed and effective professional- and personal-development decisions for themselves. It also ensures that career issues in both micro (personal, within an institution) and macro (national, cross-sector, international) career environments are taken into consideration.

PRACTICAL TOOLS

Cultural Transition Workshops and Welcome Kits

(Adapted from Tech Valley Connect's programs and resources for both new hires and employers.)

Three workshop sessions of 2 h each address critical topics for successful integration into US national and New York regional cultures, as indicated below.

Session 1. United States Culture, Customs and Traditions

- US history overview
- Encountering cultural differences
- Business etiquette/social subtleties
- Household (grocery stores; school culture; helping children transition and cope with cultural issues; understanding free speech after the 9/11 events)

Session 2. Need to Know

- Introduction to regional ethnic affinity groups and resources
- Financials (US banking; understanding credit history and how to build one; international exchange)
- Insurance (home; auto and issues of defensive driving in snow: what to keep in the car for emergencies; helpful entities such as the American Automobile Association; emergency closings of schools, roads, etc.)

Session 3. Municipalities

- Emergency services and information (urgent care locations; police; fire)
- Health care (hospitals; physician groups and specialty affiliations; medical professionals and identifying your needs; insurance)
- The court system (traffic violations; US civil rights)
- Laws/government (political correctness; sensitivity post 9/11; taxes such as home, sales, school, income; seat belts; cell phones; corporal punishment; traffic and pedestrian ordinances)
- Language skills (covered in three additional seminars: "Talk Like a Local; Sign up ASAP!", "Adding a US Accent", and "Capital Region Geography, Restaurants and Shopping")

Welcome kits and a monthly newcomer's almanac and English practice work sheets include
Brochures with overviews on

- Finding a home in the United States
- Telephones in the United States
- Using the US medical system
- Buying or leasing a car in the United States
- US culture and history on videotape
- Connecting to the world

Laminated cards and charts provide additional useful information:

- Trouble on the road—what to do if a police officer stops you or if you have an accident
- Clothing-sizes conversions
- Restaurant vocabulary and tip chart
- Metric measurement converter
- American holidays (meaning, observation, what is closed)
- Cooking in an American kitchen (measurements, temperatures, etc.)
- Emergencies card (directions in both English and the native language to use when calling for emergency services)

Critical Areas to Cover in Helping Individuals Navigate the Complex Events and Decisions that Shape their Professional Development

(Adapted from Portia, Ltd's Scenario Toolkit to assist scientists in career decision making.)

In preparation for scenario-building workshops, participants are directed to consider in depth the following topics (among others) as applied to themselves and their career and life:

- Degree of intellectual independence (are new research questions addressed?)
- Selection of research topics after PhD (suggested by colleagues/ collaborators, self-selected, long-term interests, no clear interests, no new topic, and/or expanding PhD topic)
- Job positions since PhD (research related, not research related)
- Resources needed for research (high, low, medium)
- Resource access problems (never, sometimes, always)
- Time problems (never, always, sometimes)
- Time for research (enough/not enough)
- Internal grants (available/not available)
- External grants (early career, advanced)
- Collaborative projects (national, international, interdisciplinary)
- Publications (peer reviewed, single author, collaborative)
- Project proposals (written, submitted, successful)
- Role in projects (principal investigator, associate, assistant)
- Grant proposals (national, international)
- Number of regular collaborators
- Number of professional networks
- Membership on committees (internal/external/status)
- Membership on advisory/decision panels
- Involvement in peer review
- Editorial roles
- Public-engagement activities
- Organization of scientific conferences
- Membership on scientific committees
- Time spent in teaching (pedagogic contributions/course level)
- Work/life issues (children, unemployment, mobility)

Child Care and Dependent Care in Professional Contexts

http://dx.doi.org/10.1016/B978-0-12-800215-5.00005-1

It is not very practical having children at the moment, given that young research-
ers need to publish heaps in their first years in order to get a permanent position
one day. It's especially difficult for women. **—A woman working in astron-**
omy, age 26–35 years, married/partnered, Chile

I am exceptionally happy where I am, and would need to uproot my family
to move; with a school-going child and elderly parents, this is not an option.
—A woman working in biological sciences, age 46–55 years, married/
partnered, South Africa

For professionals in science, technology, engineering, and mathematics fields, productive interactions with individuals from their own specific disciplines should be an ongoing and career-long endeavor. From
the earliest years of graduate training, professional meetings are the
locus for both recognition of subject matter achievement and dialogue
with peers who are experts in the same field. A scientist is likely to move
through a series of institutions during a career trajectory, but the body of
scholarly work will be judged by those from within the specialty. That
specialty, and the accompanying disciplinary settings in which experts
gather, will remain a centrally important and constant factor in career
success. As society completes the shift away from the traditional social
model of male breadwinners and at-home female caregivers, changing
the culture of institutions and organizations in which scientists work is
therefore essential.

It is thus also imperative to devote effort to transforming the culture
of disciplinary endeavors so that both women and men are viewed as
both full professional colleagues and as parents and caregivers with
shared family responsibilities. Furthermore, attendance at professional
meetings is a key part of networking within the community and a source
of professional support for scientists in smaller, more isolated environments. As the Elsevier Foundation formulated plans for its initiation of
the New Scholars program, a clear priority was to support some projects
that would enable scientists to attend conferences, meetings, workshops,
and symposia by helping them arrange and/or pay for child care and
other family responsibilities. Following are three case studies of professional societies that recognized the importance of influencing the culture of their own scientific fields through deployment of family-friendly
strategies.

Case study 6 describes the efforts of a multinational life sciences society to provide on-site child care at annual meetings. The project leaders had factored in numerous obstacles to successful implementation,
but the ultimate outcome was different from that originally anticipated.
On-site child care was not feasible, but that finding stimulated the society

to identify other effective means of assessing and meeting the needs of its parent-attendees.

Case study 7 provides information on the approach taken by a physical sciences society to provide grants directly to parents and/or caregivers rather than to support on-site child care. A major outcome of the project was a deeper understanding of the specific caregiving needs of the meeting attendees and identification of more useful ways to address those needs. Subgroups of the society have tailored this family-friendly support program to suit the demographics of their particular subspecialty meetings.

Case study 8 highlights another child care grants program offering financial support to cover expenses for participants at a biological society's annual meeting. After the program garnered considerable interest, the project leaders refined their procedural guidelines for greater efficiency. More importantly, they retained considerable flexibility in how recipients with caregiving needs could deploy the support offered.

CASE STUDY 6. CHILD CARE AT THE EUROPEAN MOLECULAR BIOLOGY ORGANIZATION MEETING

Implementing organization: The European Molecular Biology Organization, Heidelberg, Germany (2008 Elsevier Foundation New Scholars Grant Awardee).

Project leaders: Gerlind Wallon, PhD and Suzanne Beveridge.

Rationale and Goals

Since 2001, the European Molecular Biology Organization (EMBO) has placed a particular focus on gender balance. The organization has pioneered many actions in support of women and families, particularly with regard to conditions for postdoctoral fellows and young investigators. Each year the organization publishes gender-disaggregated statistics regarding the participation of female scientists in EMBO's activities, and has published a landmark study regarding the success rate of female applicants to EMBO's postdoctoral fellowships and young investigator program.[41] This study showed that traditional gender roles and family responsibilities are one of the key reasons why the careers of young women scientists do not progress as rapidly as those of their male peers. Other studies have shown that women attend fewer conferences and meetings, thereby foregoing the opportunities for exposure and networking.[37]

A challenge for scientists with families—and particularly those early in their careers whose studies and career moves generally take them away from traditional family-support networks—is ensuring that children are cared for while parents attend scientific conferences. Participation in such conferences offers significant opportunities for young scientists to advance their careers through education, presentations, and networking. In support of scientist-parents, EMBO offered child care at its large, annual pan-European life sciences conference. Child care by a team of professional caregivers was offered for children from 6 months up to 14 years of age.

Project Description and Outcomes

EMBO organizes an annual life science congress, The EMBO Meeting.[42] The series was started in 2009 following the European Life Scientist Organization meeting as a counterpart to the large annual meetings taking place in the United States. The EMBO Meeting is attended by approximately 1500 participants from around the world and its program reflects science of the highest quality. The meeting offers scientists from all areas of the life sciences the opportunity to hear from leaders in the field of molecular biology. Child care was offered at The EMBO Meeting in 2009 (Amsterdam), 2010 (Barcelona), and 2011 (Vienna).

In the pilot year, a number of challenges were considered before determining how best to provide on-site child care for conference participants.[43] Caregivers needed to be multilingual, as children were expected from many different language backgrounds. Nevertheless, the number of languages that could be covered was limited. A broad range of ages was envisioned, with the program catering to the needs of children aged 6 months to 14 years. On-site facilities were planned, so that the conference venue would serve as a base for the service, as were appropriate catering and access to public transportation. Finally, it was decided that care would not be restricted to safekeeping; rather, the children would have a fulfilling day with a program that sparked their imagination.

In discussions with members of the scientific community during the planning stage, EMBO found that they were extremely positive about the prospect of on-site conference child care. All scientists addressed found the offer a necessary and excellent step toward the creation of equal opportunity, and appreciated consideration of the needs of scientist-parents. EMBO then contracted with a child care service provider with a fluency in three languages who had experience in caring for children with multilingual backgrounds, as well as a team that could meet specific requirements as needed. In addition, this provider had the necessary flexibility to react on short notice to changes in requirements that emerged during the registration phase. The team of caregivers hired consisted initially of four persons plus a support team of two. On short notice, the team was able to cover Italian-speaking children in addition to those who spoke English, German, French, and Spanish at the meeting in Amsterdam.

For the first year of child care at an EMBO meeting (Amsterdam, 2009), nine children, aged 3–13 years and speaking five languages, were registered. The child care room was located close to the conference lecture rooms, allowing fast and easy access for the parents. The room was equipped with desks and chairs provided by the conference center and mattresses and materials for play provided by the child care team. Food and drink were catered by the conference center. The venue had a direct entrance into a large family park area and was only a tram ride away from the city center. This arrangement permitted the children to spend most of their time exploring the city or playing in the park and its playgrounds.

In the second year of the program (Barcelona, 2010), 12 children, aged 2–10 years, were enrolled in the program. Rooms were rented on the conference site, and catering was provided by the conference catering service in consultation with the child care provider. Children were offered age-appropriate programs. An additional room allowed parents with children under 18 months old to change diapers, put the children to sleep, or feed them in a quiet place. The conference site had a beautiful garden/park where the children could play. Easy access to public transit facilitated exploration of the city by the older children (accompanied by adults), who as a consequence saw more of the city than did their parents.

For the third year of the program (Vienna, 2011), 16 parents initially expressed an interest in the child care services, but at the actual meeting, only four children under the age of 2 years were registered. A babysitting service was offered to the parents at the rate of 20 Euros per hour, with EMBO contributing 160 Euros per child and covering the accommodation costs of the care provider.

Implementation Highlights

The child care service itself worked extremely well. Key to the success of the service provided to children and parents was a competent and reliable child care team that, as an added challenge in Europe, had to be multilingual. A team was hired that was able to follow the conference throughout Europe during the three years of the project, such that experience gained at one meeting would not be lost at the next conference site. From the beginning, the goal of the child care service was to offer a program that would be fun, entertaining, and educational for the children. Older children explored the city or visited science museums or aquariums, while younger children went to playgrounds and nearby parks. Handicraft activities rounded out the program. Feedback from parents and children alike was strongly positive in this regard. Having child care space rented on-site at the conferences provided a home base from which to start activities. These rooms were also used by parents of small children who did not otherwise take advantage of the formal child care program.

Lessons Learned

Even when the child care service was offered for free, the number of participating children was significantly lower than originally projected when meeting attendees were surveyed about their needs. There was no significant increase in use over the course of the three years that the service was offered. Despite notifications sent via e-mail to conference participants, advertisement on the meeting Web sites, and enhanced publicity about the service at the later meetings, many participants said that they were not aware of the offer of child care. Many who had initially expressed an interest subsequently responded that they had found an alternative solution for child care at home.

While an in-depth analysis was not conducted on the reasons why parents did not use the service, anecdotal evidence collected from meeting participants did indicate a number of factors. First, alternative solutions at home seemed to be preferable due (mostly) to the children's familiarity with those caregivers. There were also significant financial costs associated with travel and accommodations for children, as well as overlap with school days. Second, the inconvenience of having to take care of children in the evenings inhibited the ability of parents to participate in significant networking opportunities, one of the reasons for attending a general meeting in the first place.

On the other hand, the services offered were excellent both from the point of view of the activities offered to the children and the proficiency and flexibility of the caregivers. A local child care service would have been difficult to identify from the onset and most likely could not have offered the necessary breadth of languages. In addition, lessons learned from previous years would have been largely lost, as each year a new provider would have had to create the experience anew. It appears that parents with younger children seem to have a greater need for this type of on-site child care. A number of parents attended the meetings with smaller children (younger than 3 years old). For this reason, the qualifying age for children to be eligible for child care was decreased during the program to 9 months and a room for parents with babies was offered.

However, the on-site catering at the large conference facilities was not easily adapted to children's needs. Mainly, portions were too big, the service was not flexible regarding timing and feedback, and the meals could be extremely costly.

Sustainability

In general, the project demonstrated that on-site child care services at these particular scientific meetings are not a sustainable activity. For the service to be self-sustaining, a minimum of 30 children would need to be registered at a charge of 45 Euros per child per day. Based on the experience from three sequential annual meetings, attaining that number of participating children is highly unlikely.

Conclusions

On-site child care, even when aimed at under-school-aged children, does not seem to be a sustainable activity for this particular annual meeting. EMBO may in the future continue to offer on-site babysitting services, the costs of which are to be covered mostly by the parents, with limited grants to be provided by EMBO. As an alternative, EMBO may look for funding to provide grants to scientist-parents to finance extra child care costs incurred while these parents are participating in The EMBO Meeting. Given EMBO's current experience and feedback from other professional societies, about 15–20 applications would be anticipated annually. Such a level of interest would involve amounts of between 200 and 500 Euros as eligible costs per applicant, requiring about 7500 euros per year in total support.

CASE STUDY 7. CHILD CARE AT THE AMERICAN PHYSICAL SOCIETY ANNUAL MEETINGS

Implementing organization: Committee on the Status of Women in Physics of the American Physical Society, College Park, Maryland, USA (2008 Elsevier Foundation New Scholars Grant Awardee).
Project leaders: Mary Hall Reno, PhD, and Theodore Hodapp, PhD.

Rationale and Goals

The Committee on the Status of Women in Physics (CSWP), on behalf of the American Physical Society (APS), is committed to supporting attendance by young families/caregivers at the large APS annual meetings. Addressing the challenge of managing family responsibilities is a key area in which professional societies, such as APS, can support the diversity of their membership. The CSWP program supported early-career women, as well as men, working in physics who needed assistance with child care expenses—such as the costs of caring for an accompanying child or those incurred for extra child care at home while the parent is away—associated with attending the APS annual March or April meeting. One of the goals was to increase awareness of the importance of child care assistance in the physics and broader science communities. Another, broader goal was to influence the culture of the science field, which is shifting away from a traditional model that assumes a male breadwinner to one in which parents share family responsibilities.

Project Description and Outcomes

CSWP and APS expanded a pilot initiative that had provided funds to young attendees of the APS annual meetings in order to help create a more family-friendly environment at these meetings, with an ultimate goal of attracting and retaining more women into the field of physics. With grants of up to $400, men and women had the opportunity to cover child care-related expenses associated with attendance at the APS annual meetings. The March meeting now attracts more than 8000 attendees and the April meeting, almost 1500. These meetings include plenary talks for all attendees and concurrent sessions featuring short talks to smaller groups. In many subfields, the smaller sessions are an early opportunity for young researchers to present their work. Attendance at these meetings is a key part of networking within the physics community and a source of professional support for physicists in smaller, more isolated environments. In general, participation at such meetings is considered to be a prerequisite for career advancement.

Between 2009 and 2011, child care reimbursement requests from 89 potential attendees of the APS spring meetings were reviewed by a subcommittee of the CSWP, with priority being given to physicists at early stages of their careers. During this time, APS committed $15,000 in funds ($5000 per year) to match the Elsevier grant funding. Over the 3-year funding period, APS awarded 79 child care grants to APS Spring meeting attendees, 47 of whom were graduate students or postdoctoral associates and 21 of whom were pretenure or early-career academics.

Implementation Highlights

Child care grants are an excellent alternative to offering an on-site day care center. In the past, the APS has made efforts to help its members during meetings by offering on-site child care. This service was underutilized and, as a result, is no longer offered. The APS continues, however, to set aside spaces near scientific sessions as parent–child quiet rooms, which are occasionally used by nursing mothers in addition to parents with older children. Utilization of the parent–child quiet rooms is still sparse and, at some meetings, expensive (costs include furniture, drinking fountain rental, etc.). A CSWP subcommittee is exploring this situation and its sustainability. Overall, however, child care grants have been a huge success for APS, yielding increased use of resources as well as lowered costs and liability for the organization.

Lessons Learned

Between the first and second years of the program, there was a 47% increase in the number of applications for child care grants, likely the result of additional advertising in APS publications and via LISTSERVs and word of mouth.[44] The program also received publicity in *Nature*, a leading weekly international scientific journal, which heightened the child care grants program's visibility in the science community at large and likely contributed to the increase in applications.[45] In the first year of the child care grant program, all grant recipients were awarded the full $400 grant. Because several recipients did not utilize the entire award amount (and had staff been better informed of the applicants' needs), more grants could have been awarded. Staff, therefore, began to request applicants to estimate the dollar amount needed for their child care expenses. This approach allowed for more grants to be approved. Because of both greater publicity and more efficient cost allocations, the number of grants approved increased 42% from 2009 to 2011.

Sustainability

Following the success of the child care grants at the two national APS meetings, four APS divisions (Fluid Dynamics, Particles and Fields, Plasma Physics, and Physics of Beams) have initiated similar child care grant programs for their meetings. About 10 additional APS divisions, sections, and topical groups have also expressed interest in participating in the program, but funding is a concern for them. APS has committed $5000/year to sustain the current program at the APS national meetings, and the CSWP has created a subcommittee to explore continuing and expanding the child care grant program.

Conclusions

The APS expects that, as this program is expanded to more meetings and as costs associated with child care rise, use of these resources will increase. The increase in utilization of the grants from 2009 to 2011 shows that the child care grant program is now "up to speed" for the national meetings, providing a new opportunity to seek more sustainable funding. As noted, one of APS's goals is to increase awareness of the importance of child care assistance in the physics and broader science communities, thus continuing to influence the culture of a scientific field that is shifting from a traditional model to a more egalitarian one.

CASE STUDY 8. CHILD CARE AT THE AMERICAN SOCIETY FOR CELL BIOLOGY ANNUAL MEETINGS

Implementing organization: Women in Cell Biology of the American Society for Cell Biology, Bethesda, Maryland, USA (2007 Elsevier Foundation New Scholars Grant Awardee).

Project leaders: Sandra K. Masur, PhD; Ursula W. Goodenough, PhD; Joan Goldberg, PhD; and Elizabeth Marincola, MBA.

Rationale and Goals

To help remove an obstacle to the professional advancement of women in cell biology, the Women in Cell Biology group proposed to establish a competitive and sustainable system for providing child care that would allow qualified cell biologists to attend a very important vehicle for career advancement, the American Society for Cell Biology (ASCB) Annual Meeting.

Project Description and Outcomes

The original proposal drew upon studies of the "leaky pipeline" for women in science and the finding that women attend fewer meetings, with the attendant loss of scientific and networking benefits for their career development. Fiona Watt, an eminent cell biologist, has enumerated "challenges for women cell biologists past and present", all of which can be seen to address this leaky pipeline.[46] These challenges included increasing the proportion of women in the most senior academic positions; the representation of women on editorial boards, conference programs, and committees that handle appointments and funding; the number of women who win prizes and are elected to national academies; and the number of women in leadership roles. Because many of these challenges are addressed by the significant opportunities for science-career development offered at ASCB's annual meeting, it is essential for young female cell biologists to be able to participate fully in these meetings. A common barrier to their participation at this crucial stage in their careers is the absence of child care. The lack of financial support for child care in association with meeting attendance is a significant component of this barrier.

The ASCB project had two objectives. The first was to develop and implement a Child Care Award for attendees to remove an obstacle to participation in the major meeting of cell biologists. The approach chosen was to provide the financial assistance that would allow for individualized solutions. ASCB staff would administer the awards program and oversee the work of ASCB volunteers from the Women in Cell Biology Committee to establish criteria and serve on the recipient-selection committee. The second objective was to facilitate the establishment of permanent support programs at member institutions. This approach required compensation for 25% of an ASCB staff person's time so that he or she could make a significant commitment to establishing such a permanent program by building relationships with financial/administrative officers at member institutions and with the local organizing committee for each annual meeting.

To develop and implement the Child Care Award, ASCB engaged in the following activities from 2008 to 2010: (1) establishing criteria for the award, (2) designing an application form, (3) selecting an awards committee, (4) advertising the child care awards, (5) reviewing applications (performed by the awards committee), (6) selecting winners and announcing the awards, and (7) disseminating the funding at the ASCB annual meeting. In the first year, 14 of 19 applicants received awards; in the second year, 15 of 16 applicants did; and in the third year, 33 of 44 applicants did. For the fourth year of the program (2011), 30 of 31 applicants received Child Care Awards. The awards clearly made an impact on awardees in that they supported their attendance at an important meeting and affirmed that being a parent is not at odds with being a fully engaged scientist.

Implementation Highlights

The ASCB was unable to conduct the second objective of the project, reaching out to member institutions to establish similar programs, due to resource constraints. However, the child care grants program facilitating scientific meeting attendance clearly worked well. For many individuals, applying for and receiving the grant provided a model of the type of resources that could support their career development when they are faced with competing pressures in work and life.

All grantees were required to present abstracts at the meeting, thus motivating them to further their careers through presentation of their science. The meeting also offered extensive opportunities for networking and interaction with other scientists, including poster sessions held throughout its duration.

Critical to the implementation of the program was having an award and a grant application that were both "user friendly". These two elements were seen as crucial to optimizing the cost-benefit of the awards: coverage of reasonable costs and ease of application. The first criterion was met by allowing the grants to cover any reasonable child care arrangement. The ASCB explicitly stated that it would pay for a caretaker at home; for a relative or caretaker to travel to one's home; for children to travel to a relative; to retain child care at the site of the annual meeting; for extended day care hours; or to bring a caretaker (related or not) to accompany the parent (especially a nursing mother) to the meeting. There was also an "other" category leaving open the possibility that there may be creative and legitimate child care solutions that parent-applicants wish to propose.

The second criterion required that the application itself not be, or be perceived as, a barrier to seeking help. By definition, those applying have limited time, so ASCB sought to eliminate requests for unnecessary data. The application is basic: "Tell us how many children you have; how old they are; how you would apply the money if granted; and how much you are requesting." The only "research" required of the applicant was a requirement to provide an accurate estimate of travel costs (independently verified by the committee). The application was estimated to take 15–20 min to complete.

Very clear and stage-appropriate criteria for selection of awardees were established by the Award Selection Committee; information about these criteria was also requested on the application. The criteria required the applicant to be an ASCB member (easily accomplished); submit an abstract to the annual meeting; provide a reasonable estimate of travel costs, if needed; and prove need. Examples of such need included someone who is breast-feeding and must bring the child; is a single parent; or is a member of a two-parent household but where the second parent cannot care for the child and additional child care costs will be accrued. Other need scenarios include both parents are attending the meeting and both are presenting posters, so additional child care is required; additional child care costs will be incurred at home because the parent(s) will not be available after normal child care hours; additional costs will be incurred to bring both the child and a caregiver to the meeting; and additional costs will be incurred to bring a relative to the home to care for the child.

Lessons Learned

Financial support to pay for child care during the ASCB meeting made it possible for people to attend this important scientific conference each year. Specifically, the design of the award allowed each candidate to craft an individualized solution that worked best for both parent(s) and child(ren). Thus awardees could propose to use the funds to pay for a caregiver at home, for a caregiver's travel to the meeting, for child care at the convention site, or for another appropriate use that met the award criteria. Importantly, the awardees felt validated by the leaders of their chosen field, cell biology. The award confirmed their potential to make significant scientific contributions and for advancement at a time when they face multiple challenges to their confidence that they will be able to persevere and succeed.

Another insight was that advertising an award is necessary but not sufficient to bring it to the attention of the very busy people at whom the information is aimed. Placing an article in the ASCB newsletter highlighting the program (just prior to the deadline for submitting abstracts) more than doubled the number of applicants. The timing of the article and the more extensive information it provided, in addition to placement of multiple advertisements about the grants, contributed to the increase in the number of competitive applicants.

Sustainability

The ASCB developed a well-received and well-reviewed child care awards program with clear, verifiable criteria, designed a simple and effective application, selected an awards committee, experimented with ways to advertise the awards, reviewed applications, and disseminated this critical funding at its annual meeting. The simplicity of the program and its success, demonstrated by its increasing use by its target audience and testimonials over 3 years, provided the organization with confirmation that it offers an attractive and proven package to present for future philanthropic support.

Conclusions

The ASCB Child Care Awards program presents a model that should be easy to emulate. The program and its guidelines could be easily adopted and adapted by other organizations. The opportunity to develop the program and test it over 3 years allowed for verification of the need for the child care award and provided sufficient data to attract funding to continue the program at the ASCB.[47,48]

PRACTICAL TOOLS

Model Application for Child Care Support

(Adapted from the American Society for Cell Biology initiative.)

Applicant Contact Information

* Abstract acceptance no.:	* City:
* Abstract title:	* State/province:
* First name:	* Zip/postal code:
* Last name:	* Country:
* Institution:	* Phone:
* Department:	* Fax:
* Address:	* E-mail:

Application Questions

1. Funds may be applied to the following needs.
   a. Home-based child care expenses incurred because of ASCB Annual Meeting attendance (funds may not be applied to normal ongoing expense). Please indicate the city and state, and if not the US, country where you reside:
   b. Travel of a relative or other care provider to my home to care for my child(ren) while I attend the ASCB Annual Meeting. Please indicate where the provider is traveling to/from:
   c. Travel of my child(ren) to the location of a care provider who does not live in my community. Please indicate where the child(ren) will be cared for (city/state/country if not US):
   d. Travel of a care provider to the ASCB Annual Meeting with me to care for my child(ren) in that city. Please indicate where the provider will be traveling from:
   e. Child care to be retained on-site at the Annual Meeting.
   f. Other (please explain):
2. My anticipated dates of attendance at the ASCB Annual Meeting are from (mm/dd/yyyy) to (/ /)
3. I am a:

PhD student	Senior faculty member or late-career scientist
Postdoctoral fellow	Other (please specify):
Junior faculty member or early-career independent scientist	

4. My child(ren) will be the following age(s) as of December 18, 2013:
5. Please indicate to the Child care Grant Selection Committee the circumstances that prompt you to request this award. Please explain circumstances if the other parent cannot assume child care responsibilities. (350 character limit)

6. The anticipated expenses indicated above are (please itemize):
    Travel (for whom, and to/from):
    Child care expenses (caregiver, dates, and approximate total cost):
    Other (specify):

Total estimated cost:
Total funds requested from ASCB:

Promoting Family-Friendly Policies

Equitable Solutions for Retaining a Robust STEM Workforce.
http://dx.doi.org/10.1016/B978-0-12-800215-5.00006-3

There is not a policy for supporting family members at my institution. **—A man working in life sciences, age 46–55 years, married/partnered, Brazil**

I am working part time, only two days a week, so I can spend most of my time with my daughter (who is a toddler). **—A woman working in earth and planetary sciences, age 26–35 years, married/partnered, USA**

Academic institutions can occupy highly visible leadership roles in addressing the needs of their employees, especially faculty members and earlier career stage scientists. Like the organizations and professional societies profiled in Chapters 3, 4, and 5, academia is obligated to take significant responsibility for meeting the challenges of dual-career households and of scientists who are parents and caregivers. For science, technology, engineering, and mathematics (STEM) faculty and scholars, it is essential to recognize their need for professional travel and conference attendance. Although many women face the challenge of starting a family just at the time they are hitting stride in their professional careers, the impact of this transition on women in STEM is especially pronounced—particularly in academia. Many of the factors discouraging women from entering the higher academic faculty ranks and leadership positions in STEM fields are directly related to institutional climate and the difficulty of balancing work and home responsibilities. Unfortunately, due to the nature of higher education, a single approach will not meet the needs of all academic institutions. This chapter presents four case studies of Elsevier New Scholars projects in which universities have successfully grappled with creating a more female-focused, dual-career oriented, and family-friendly institution.

Case study 9 presents the work of a state university that led a five-institution consortium in developing programs to address the career-development needs of their faculty members. The primary focus was on removal of travel-related barriers to the professional advancement of STEM researchers with child care and dependent care responsibilities, particularly women and dual-career couples. Men with dependent care responsibilities were also included. Networking approaches and outreach to professional societies and granting agencies were also part of the project, in order to promote further the strategies that assist female scientists in their career advancement.

Case study 10 features a large state university that implemented a three-part program of awards for travel child care or elder care, matching support funds for active service-modified duties (ASMD), and information about family-friendly policies and programs for early-career female scholars in STEM fields. Publicizing the success of the programs for more widespread implementation across the institution's schools and departments was also an important part of the project.

Case study 11, set at a private university, describes a project focused on the postdoctoral period to address two key needs related to professional travel: a dependent care program for postdoctoral fellows and travel support for fellows whose spouses were graduate students or postdoctoral fellows in science and engineering at another institution. The focus on the postdoctoral period was an essential element of this particular project, because a disproportionate number of women researchers at the postdoctoral career stage opt out of future assistant professor positions at research universities.

Case study 12 describes a state university that addressed work/life support issues after junior faculty returned to work following the birth or adoption of a child. Two connected initiatives were a feature of the project: creation of a lactation policy and program for new breast-feeding mothers returning to the workplace and an education and awareness initiative for the broader university community about work/life issues in general.

CASE STUDY 9. THE FAMILY TRAVEL INITIATIVE

Implementing organization: University of Massachusetts-Amherst, Amherst, Massachusetts, USA (2009 Elsevier Foundation New Scholars Grant Awardee.)

Project leaders: Maria Santore, PhD; Rebecca Spencer, PhD; and Barbara Pearson, PhD.

Rationale and Goals

The focus of this project was the removal of travel-related barriers to the professional advancement of STEM researchers with child care and dependent care responsibilities. An overall goal was to promote women and dual-career couples; men with dependent care responsibility were also included in the target group. The project served the Five Colleges (University of Massachusetts-Amherst, aka UMass Amherst; Smith College; Mount Holyoke College; Amherst College; and Hampshire College), as well as faculty and postdoctoral researchers from across the country.

The approach had four facets: education, travel support (financial), advocacy to professional societies and granting agencies, and networking (to identify and share resources). While the immediate objectives of the STEM Family Travel Initiative (FTI) targeted the advancement of faculty and postdoctoral researchers in STEM departments at UMass Amherst and within the Five College system, STEM FTI also aimed to catalyze cultural change at the national level. A system was envisioned in which professional societies offer affordable on-site child care at meetings; user facilities (such as national laboratories with X-ray and neutron instrumentation) have reserved, drop-in child care space at nearby accredited centers; granting agencies and universities allow budget line items to cover travel-related child care; and these same agencies have a mechanism in place to allow scientists with dependent care responsibilities to participate fully in panels and workshops, many of which are requirements on grants. While these long-term cultural goals were not expected to be realized in the near term, the STEM FTI targeted specific components of this vision to bring the goals closer to realization.

Project Description and Outcomes

The expansion and maintenance of an interactive Web site was a critical educational aspect of the project. It allowed users (in the Five Colleges and beyond) to access and learn about all facets of the program.[49] The Web site includes an explanation of STEM FTI's mission, applications for travel-support awards, announcements of educational programs and summaries of past workshops, updated listings of professional societies offering child care and how to access these services, and a survey targeting national-level input on the degree of interest in on-site child care at professional meetings of relatively large societies. Links to the STEM FTI Web site from the Faculty Development and Human Resources Departments at each of the Five Colleges were put in place. Links to and from professional societies to the Web site, especially the survey on the need for child care at national meetings, were also a critical aspect of this networking activity. The Web site has been maintained so that all information is current, especially regarding programs and deadlines for child care-related programs at professional societies. The site's professional society page now reports on 12 different professional societies, with expansion of the list expected as interest in the program grows. Links to federal agency Web sites, when relevant, were also included. For example, National Institutes of Health policy affects professional meetings in that organizers utilizing NIH support must provide information about child care to attendees in advance.[50]

The continually growing grant program covered incremental costs of child care during professional travel. Travel grants of up to $1200 per year for dependent care during overnight trips, and up to $150 per year in day trips were made available to tenure-track faculty and postdoctoral associates within STEM departments at the Five Colleges. During the 3-year duration of the project (2010–2012), awards were granted to 49 individuals, 33 of whom were women. While most recipients were faculty members, nine of the awards were to postdoctoral scholars. The awards went to individuals at Smith College, Hampshire College, Mount Holyoke College, Amherst College, and the University of Massachusetts.

Workshops targeted to faculty, postdoctoral fellows, and graduate students were held as part of the program. The first was on the importance of travel to the professional advancement of academics, with specific attention paid to the relatively high level of travel implicitly required of junior faculty working in the areas of materials, biomaterials, physics, and chemistry. The years prior to the tenure decision were emphasized. A second topical workshop, electronically networked to Five College faculty via Skype, addressed the challenges of traveling with children and solicited feedback to the STEM FTI on areas where participants thought networking and travel support were critical. These education programs were later extended beyond the Five College institutions to venues at relevant professional societies.

Several program grantees were given the opportunity to participate on work/life panels sponsored by professional society conference committees, at which they were able to explain how STEM FTI works and to encourage society members to advocate for similar programs at their own institutions. To enhance this new avenue of education and advocacy, a third workshop bridging education and advocacy for Five College travelers was formulated. In this program, a small group of travelers met to brainstorm about leveraging these new opportunities and to design materials to help people make optimal use of them. Some of the ideas they generated were translated into additional STEM FTI initiatives. In 2012, a workshop was held to explain the new backup child care available to the campus community. There were presentations by representatives of Parents in a Pinch (a temporary nanny/sitter placement agency), University Human Resources, and STEM FTI, all of which aimed to increase awareness of the new benefit, which is now provided uniformly to all University of Massachusetts (nonstudent) employees.[51]

To provide additional support on the child care front, the university offered free membership to the national Web-based babysitting bulletin board SitterCity to its faculty. For faculty at the other four of the Five Colleges, these fees were covered by the STEM FTI grants. While this resource was initially underutilized, its positive impact has increased. One concern that continues to resonate at STEM FTI workshops is that, in addition to the large monetary expense of travel-related child care (and related travel expenses for children and/or providers), making arrangements for such care is daunting when on-site care is not available. STEM FTI has therefore provided resources for travelers through a number of other routes, such as working with the UMass Amherst administration to make Sitter-City available as a benefit of employment. While the original intent of the project was to develop a parents' network and database of providers, this approach was unlikely to succeed because large numbers of academic travelers relied on family rather than hired sitters for child care. Many academic travelers indicated, however, that they would consider using drop-in care at established day care centers near travel destinations for their school-aged and preschool-aged children. They also felt that having a list of resources would be useful. This was a desirable option because established centers are insured and frequently (but not always) regulated by the states in which they reside.

In 2011, the project abandoned the original plan to provide a parents' network based on academic travel to different cities; feedback continues to suggest this was a wise choice. Instead, the program currently maintains a roster of facilities in five cities that regularly host technical conferences at their convention centers, as well as facilities in the regions near the National Science Foundation, National Institutes of Health, and the National Institute of Standards and Technology. Candidate day care centers were identified within a 5-mile radius of each destination (the conference center within each city, or the agency itself). Those centers were polled to determine if they would offer short-term drop-in care to academic travelers; the program then created and now maintains a list of those that do. This list is available to STEM FTI travelers, but is not posted on the Web site because of rapidly changing policies at individual centers. The program also offers to do the research for interested Five College faculty on child care centers within a certain radius of other meeting locations, but does not provide formal recommendations for any of the specific centers so identified.

Another strategy adopted to mitigate the burden of finding reliable child care for academic travelers was to engage a formal nanny/babysitting network with a company that uses its own providers. (This option differs from vehicles such as SitterCity, which are simply electronic forums on which to advertise and which leave the job of interviewing, selecting, and ensuring reliability to the parent/traveler.) In 2011, STEM FTI contacted the UMass Amherst administration to convey the need for reliable, insured child sitting coverage for its employees. As a result of a meeting between leaders at UMass Amherst and Parents in a Pinch (see above), the university signed a formal contract with the agency, in which the parameters of need for traveling academics are addressed such that the program provides the necessary support for traveling parents and caregivers. The contract provides 20 days of usage per year per employee, effective in both the local area and major conference cities. Critical implementation details are a responsibility of the University's Human Resources Department. At least one other institution among the Five Colleges (Mount Holyoke) negotiated a contract with Parents in a Pinch for its own campus. The availability of this type of child care support represents a great advance not only in accommodating the need for emergency care locally, but also in serving academic travelers by making licensed and insured sitters available through one phone call or e-mail in most major cities where faculty and postdoctoral researchers are likely to travel. Current statistics suggest moderate use of this resource in its first year, with about 15% of the usage occurring outside of Amherst and 20% devoted to elder care. In January 2013, the contract with Parents in a Pinch was renewed for a second year, providing a continued benefit to travelers and faculty in need of short-term dependent care support in the Amherst area and beyond. Its popularity is expected to grow with additional advertising and word-of-mouth testimonials.

Advocacy to professional societies has been conducted in several ways. The goal is to raise awareness among the leadership of professional societies of the issues surrounding meeting travel and dependent care needs. In this way, STEM FTI aims to plant the seeds that will someday make possible affordable child care at large meetings. First, as part of the travel grant program, letters discussing the need for dependent care have been sent to contacts at professional societies sponsoring the conferences to which the grantees travel.[52] Additionally, discussions are ongoing with the American Chemical Society (ACS), which has a history of providing complimentary day care to meeting attendees traveling with children. Feedback from the ACS is being used to develop strategies for approaching other technical societies that do not offer this benefit to their members. A questionnaire, prominent on the STEM FTI Web site and open to all, can be used to assess the level of interest in child care at the meetings of a variety of professional societies, especially those not currently offering any type of child care. Once sufficient statistics have been collected based on answers to the questionnaire, STEM FTI will contact professional societies to inform them of the interest among their membership in on-site child care.

Importantly, a "plug and play" advocacy campaign was developed, aimed at scientists beyond the Five Colleges, in which Five College meeting attendees would introduce their peers to the program while they are at meetings, bring them to the Web site, and guide them to the questionnaires. Campaign materials include packages of cards and notes of talking points. STEM FTI leaders also identified and contacted agencies that provide bonded child care at meetings and corporate events and now maintain updated cost estimates for their services at technical meetings, establishing a starting point for professional societies interested in pursuing their own on-site child care programs.

Implementation Highlights

In the second year of development, the awards program was expanded to three review cycles per year to increase the number of applications and to reduce the possibility that academic travelers might miss an opportunity to apply due to late notice of a meeting. Because of this, a broad group of individuals from many different disciplines has been reached, including those working in life sciences, physical sciences, applied sciences, and engineering. Support was also made available to academic professionals traveling to granting agencies for workshops and panels, an important component of academic networking often translating (indirectly) to research funding. Notably, assistant professor grantees (in year one of the program) have moved through the tenure process successfully, in part because of the travel support. STEM FTI's flexibility with regard to choice of provider and child care mechanisms is an advantage rarely seen with other programs. It has been much appreciated by the travel-support awardees because it allows children to travel with the parent or stay with other family members. Child care support is also now provided for seminar speakers and faculty candidates with children who will be coming to UMass Amherst. Modest monetary support is also provided by academic departments and promoted by the university administration, and a short list is maintained of established local centers offering drop-in care.

Lessons Learned

An up-to-date Web site for providing information and interactions between various constituents proved to be essential. Similarly, formal workshops not only served as an educational vehicle, but also provided information essential to driving the next phases of the STEM FTI programs and to identifying which resources are most needed. Providing monetary travel support to a diverse body of academics is a strong concept, but to be most effective, application procedures and timing must be adjusted to best accommodate the schedules of academic travelers. In identifying and assessing child care provider networks, approaches should be adjusted to ensure efficiency and cost and time effectiveness. As noted, STEM FTI's flexibility with regard to child care mechanisms is an advantage rarely seen with other programs.

Advocacy initiatives were also critical to ensuring enhanced impact for the programs. Because there was significant interest expressed beyond the Five Colleges in obtaining child care support during meetings, the challenge now is to identify the best ways to quantify it. Meeting attendees' willingness to be verbally supportive far outweighs the likelihood of their going online and electronically expressing their interest in a quantifiable way. Such reliable statistics will be essential for making the case for expanded child care options to interested societies and, ultimately, funding agencies. To disseminate these initiatives more broadly, it will be necessary to forge partnerships with other universities to increase the user base on the surveys about child care needs at professional society meetings. It is now a goal to develop an advocacy budget to allow faculty to travel to regular technical meetings where they can present program materials at mentoring sessions.

Sustainability

Toward long-term impact and sustainability, STEM FTI has been partnering with prominent scientific centers at UMass Amherst, using them as sites for advertising the project's educational programs, travel-support grants, and advocacy activities. The centers also serve as liaisons between STEM FTI and funding agencies. STEM FTI activities have been highlighted during the outreach portions of the centers' evaluation presentations, and these funding agencies are becoming aware of the issues that individuals face in balancing dependent care and professional travel.

Advocacy activities targeting policy changes in this area can potentially be very effective, but must be approached strategically. For example, STEM FTI is seeking a change in university policy to enable reimbursement of incremental dependent care expenses resulting from business travel, thus moving these expenses into the same category as mileage or meals. This aggressive advocacy approach was inspired by the public review period for proposed changes in federal grant policies.[53] Using the same letter sent to the government's online forum, key university personnel were enlisted to participate in negotiations on the campus's indirect cost rate, to take place in 2013. The following two provisions need to be satisfied: establishment of a uniform policy for reimbursement and assurance that charges are consistent with those normally allowed by non-federal sponsors. In UMass Amherst's case, the campus subscription to Parents in a Pinch satisfies the first criterion. The challenge in meeting the second provision for nonfederal sponsors is the current language in Massachusetts state codes. As a result of outreach by university personnel, the local state representative, a long-time advocate for women's issues, plans to bring the issue before the State House Counsel, the first step before a regulatory change can proceed to the Ethics Commission. An incremental approach in this matter helps to ensure that, regardless of the immediate outcome, the number of people who recognize the importance of women's advancement in STEM disciplines will increase.

Conclusions

STEM FTI has begun the removal of travel-related barriers to the professional advancement of STEM researchers with dependent care responsibilities and in the promotion of women in STEM disciplines through education, advocacy, and support. The program has successfully provided monetary travel support to a diverse body of academics, adjusting application procedures and timing to best accommodate recipients' needs. In addition, the advocacy portion of the program has grown significantly, resulting in an expanded impact. Work continues toward the long-term goal of catalyzing cultural change on the national level.

CASE STUDY 10. ENHANCING THE ACADEMIC CLIMATE FOR WOMEN SCHOLARS THROUGH FAMILY-FRIENDLY POLICIES

Implementing organization: University of California, Los Angeles, California, USA (2009 Elsevier Foundation New Scholars Grant Awardee.)

Project leaders: Christine A. Littleton, JD, and Susan Drange Lee.

Rationale and Goals

The program, based at the University of California, Los Angeles (UCLA), had three broad objectives: (1) to identify and confront family-related barriers to women's progress in academic careers in science, health, and technology; (2) to encourage retention of women faculty in science, health, and technology by reducing the impact of workload following childbirth or adoption; and (3) to increase entry of women into academic or research careers in science, health, and technology by facilitating opportunities for those with child care responsibilities to attend professional meetings.

Project Description and Outcomes

The project consisted of three parts: travel child care awards, matching-support funds for ASMD, and informational programs about family-friendly policies and programs for female scholars in the fields of science, health, and engineering.

Travel Childcare Awards for Female Postdoctoral Scholars and Assistant Professors in Science, Health, and Technology

In an academic's life, the years immediately following completion of the doctorate and the early years pretenure are critical for gaining exposure and recognition of one's research, networking for faculty positions, and solidifying one's career objectives. These years are also women's prime childbearing years and thus are a time of a great stress and conflict for those who wish both to pursue a career in academic research and raise a family. To address this challenge, Travel Childcare Awards of $500 each were offered to defray the costs of child care, travel, and registration fees for conferences and meetings related to science, health, and technology for female postdoctoral scholars and assistant professors with child care responsibilities.[54] Applications for Travel Childcare Awards are accepted twice a year, in the fall and spring quarters. Awards are made based on need, importance of the meeting to the applicant's career, and the funding available.

Since 2010, 76 awards have been made available. Faculty and scholars in eight divisions of the institution are eligible: engineering, life sciences, physical sciences, public health, dentistry, medicine, nursing, and social sciences. The majority (64%) of support has gone to participants in medicine, with the remainder more evenly distributed across the other seven fields. The heavy utilization by participants in medicine may be related to the much larger number of assistant professors and postdoctoral scholars in medicine compared with those in the other schools and divisions, combined with more opportunities to attend conferences.

ASMD Matching Support Funds for Ladder-Rank Women Faculty in Science, Health, and Technology

Due to the need to maintain research productivity, women faculty members in the laboratory sciences often prefer working a reduced schedule to taking off full time for a quarter. This part of UCLA's program provided matching funds to assist ladder-rank women faculty members in science, health, and technology who wished to utilize the ASMD policy.[55] Through this program, a female faculty member, in conjunction with her department chair, may request a $4500 award to supplement departmental funds. These funds are to be used to enable modified or reduced duties (e.g., teaching relief and departmental service) for one academic quarter following the birth or adoption of a young child, per the University of California ASMD policy. Funds can be used to pay for a lecturer or a graduate or postdoctoral researcher to enable the faculty member to work on a reduced schedule.

Applications for the ASMD Matching Support Funds are reviewed by the Vice Provost for Diversity and Faculty Development on a rolling basis. The funds are provided based on level of need, timeliness of request, and availability of funding. Eligible schools and divisions are engineering, life sciences, physical sciences, public health, dentistry, nursing, and social sciences. In the 3 years of the program, 10 matching fund grants for ASMD were made. Utilization of this program was more evenly distributed across the schools and divisions, due mainly to the exclusion of the school of medicine from participation in this program. Because the program depends on the timing of female faculty members becoming parents, utilization varies from year to year.[54]

Balancing Work and Life as an Assistant Professor

Another program element involves increasing the dissemination of information about family-friendly policies to academic women in science, health, and engineering, as well as to department chairs, deans, and all faculty members.[56] In 2011, a panel discussion and luncheon on work/ life balance was held for assistant professors and postdoctoral scholars that highlighted issues and available resources, programs, and policies to assist in balancing work and personal life. Five prestigious senior faculty members from the departments of Electrical Engineering, Anthropology, Physics and Astronomy, Information Studies, and Rheumatology served as panelists to discuss strategies for balancing research, teaching, and service with personal commitments such as child rearing and family responsibilities. Several female vice provosts and associate deans also served as table hosts during the event. Thirty-seven faculty members attended. A special publication was also developed for the event, titled "Balancing Work and Life as an Assistant Professor". This 12-page booklet included sections on family-friendly policies, time management, resources for child care, programs for children and families, managing service commitments and sleep, exercise, and maintaining a healthy diet. It was well received and is now posted on the Faculty Diversity and Development Web site for easy access.[57]

Implementation Highlights

Overall, face-to-face meetings associated with the three-part program worked very well, while routine e-mail and Web site postings were not particularly effective in disseminating information about the program. The Childcare Travel Grants and ASMD Awards were advertised on the UCLA Faculty Diversity and Development Web site, as well as through e-mails to female postdoctoral scholars, assistant professors, associate professors, department chairs, and department administrators. The programs were also promoted in meetings with department chairs and at orientations for new faculty members and new department chairs. Stories about the programs also appeared in university publications, including articles describing the initial support for the program, the Travel Childcare Awards, and the ASMD Matching Fund programs. At the completion of the second year of this 3-year program, participation in the Travel Childcare Awards had increased. Deans agreed to endorse both the Travel Childcare Awards and the ASMD programs, and to promote them by distributing information to faculty and postdoctoral scholars in their divisions/schools.

The Assistant Professor Luncheon on Work/Life Balance was well attended and well received. Helpful strategies and tips were shared and networking connections were made among female faculty members. Based on the success of this event, another event for postdoctoral scholars and graduate students on the topic of work/life balance was held in 2012, as well as another luncheon for assistant professors on the topics of time management and balancing family responsibilities with the demands of research and professional publishing.

Lessons Learned

As with most new programs at UCLA, initial interest was somewhat slow to develop, but as word spread, an increasing number of applications for the Childcare Travel Grants were received. Another factor potentially limiting program use has to do with the general availability of travel funds at the department level. Like most academic institutions, the University of California has been making budget cuts due to reduced funding amidst difficult economic times. Funding for travel overall has been reduced, leading to fewer travel opportunities for female postdoctoral scholars and assistant professors and potentially fewer requests for assistance with child care related to such travel than would have been received in more robust economic times. In the future, program administrators will need to collaborate with units that provide underlying travel grants, such as the Academic Senate, because the travel grant covers only the additional cost attributable to child care responsibilities.

The ASMD matching fund provided four awards in its first year (2010) and one award in 2011. The level of use of the ASMD program depends on the timing of female faculty member's maternity leaves, so in some years several women are interested in utilizing this fund; in other years, fewer are. When faculty members time their childbearing to coincide with summer quarter (when most have no teaching responsibilities), they may not need to utilize ASMD, while those who give birth at other times of the year may. The greatest effect of the program has been to "normalize" ASMD, such that faculty members are more likely to request it and departments more likely to provide it, whether or not matching funding is requested.

It appears that the informational portion of the project was much needed; as part of the application process for the Childcare Travel Grant program, survey data were gathered from female postdoctoral scholars and assistant professors to assess these applicants' knowledge of various family-friendly policies at the University of California. Based on a small sample of 25, the number of respondents rating themselves as "not aware" of existing policies were as follows: 20% were not aware of the Paid/Unpaid Family Leave benefit; 32% were not aware of Tenure Clock Extension; 60% were not aware of ASMD; 72% were not aware of the Part-Time Tenure-Track Appointment; and 80% were not aware of Deferral of Appraisal (Posttenure). Such sweeping lack of awareness of existing policies speaks strongly to the importance of ongoing efforts to publicize family-friendly policies and practices within the university.

Sustainability

The interest in the Childcare Travel Grant Program has extended beyond the eligible departments and has become a model for other schools within UCLA. In 2011, both the UCLA School of Law and the Division of Humanities implemented their own Childcare Travel Grant programs, modeled after the original ones.

Changes in the administrative personnel responsible for this set of programs have made it more difficult to sustain its profile in the short term, but will create better conditions for longer term success. Both of the original principal investigators ended their terms in office in the first year of the program, but their successors enthusiastically embraced the programs and are collaborating more broadly with other administrators and faculty to assure continued activity for at least the next 5 years. The success of the programs has grown over the years, due in part to deans and department chairs endorsing and helping to promote both the Travel Childcare Awards and the ASMD programs by distributing information about them to faculty and postdoctoral scholars in their divisions/schools. In this way, awareness of the ASMD program has increased among deans and department chairs as well, fulfilling one of the goals of the project. During 2013, the intent is to create an ongoing Travel Childcare Award program, with funding provided by the deans of UCLA's schools and divisions, thereby institutionalizing this much-needed assistance for women in the early stages of their academic careers.

Conclusions

The primary success of these programs lies in the widespread acceptance of the fact that increasing the representation of women in the sciences requires acknowledgment of the additional responsibilities female faculty bear. Although responsibility for child care—and increasingly, for elder care as well—is becoming more evenly divided between spouses and partners, the change is slow and uneven. In addition, any such shifts among individual parents simply mean that institutions must pay greater attention to the needs of faculty families. The contributions of female scientists are too important to the health and vibrancy of academic institutions to allow any artificial barriers to their productivity and progress to remain unaddressed.

CASE STUDY 11. FROM GRADUATE STUDENT TO ASSISTANT PROFESSOR: HELPING POSTDOCTORAL SCIENTISTS AND ENGINEERS MEET THE DEMANDS OF CAREER AND FAMILY LIFE

Implementing organization: Princeton University, Princeton, New Jersey, USA (2007 Elsevier Foundation New Scholars Grant Awardee.) Project leader: Joan S. Girgus, PhD.

Rationale and Goals

A postdoctoral fellowship is an important stepping stone in most successful academic careers in science and engineering. The postdoctoral fellowship years are also a period of particular vulnerability in the academic career path. Large numbers of young scientists and engineers—among them a disproportionate number of women—decide at this point in their careers not to apply for assistant professor positions in the nation's research universities. There is strong evidence that the problem of balancing family and career is an important factor in the attrition seen among women researchers at this stage. Furthermore, the postdoctoral years follow directly upon that stretch of time in graduate school during which women are also particularly vulnerable, as a disproportionate number of them terminate their graduate studies before completing a PhD degree or switch their career goal from obtaining a faculty position at a research university to entering other kinds of science and engineering careers. Princeton University's overall goal is to provide the supports needed so that female (and male) graduate students, postdoctoral fellows, and faculty can flourish in both career and family life. In this particular project, focus was on the particular needs of postdoctoral scientists and engineers—which are, in some ways, different from those of either graduate students or faculty members in these fields.

Project Description and Outcomes

Over the last decade, Princeton University has developed a range of supports to make it more feasible for faculty, staff, and students—particularly women—to maintain strong trajectories in both their career and family lives. Many supports are equally useful for each of these groups. Faculty, postdoctoral fellows, and graduate students, however, have needs that are particular to their circumstances and their place along the academic career path.

First, postdoctoral fellows in science and engineering are frequently married to or in domestic partnerships with a fellow science and engineering graduate student or another postdoctoral researcher. These postdoctoral fellowship years can pose great challenges in such two-career households. It is often impossible for such couples to live together while both members pursue their best career opportunities. Furthermore, many postdoctoral appointments are for only 1 or 2 years, with the result that postdoctoral researchers often have to move at least twice in a relatively short span of time, which is especially disruptive to two-career households. Second, postdoctoral fellows and graduate students who are the parents of young children have difficulty attending academic conferences and similar career-building events—even though such events are generally acknowledged to be crucial for networking and other important career experiences—because arrangements must be made for the care of their children while the fellow or student is participating in the event.

To help talented postdoctoral fellows and graduate students at Princeton meet these challenges, two programs were developed. The first provided travel grants to postdoctoral fellows whose spouses or partners were graduate students or postdoctoral fellows in science or engineering at other institutions at some distance from Princeton, in order to mitigate the difficulties—including financial ones—caused by having to maintain separate households. The second program provided grants to pay for a wide range of child care arrangements while graduate students and postdoctoral researchers were attending academic conferences and workshops.

The Postdoctoral Spouse/Partner Travel Grant Program provided reimbursement for up to $1500 a year in travel expenses to Princeton postdoctoral fellows in the sciences and engineering who had a spouse or partner who was a full-time graduate student or postdoctoral fellow in a science or engineering field at a university at least 150 miles from Princeton. Thus, every one of these grants helped two people who were in the middle of their training as scientists or engineers; generally speaking, one of the partners was a women scientist or engineer. Twenty-nine grants were awarded to postdoctoral researchers in the natural sciences and engineering under the Spouse/Partner Travel Program. Twenty-one grants were awarded to postdoctoral researchers in the natural sciences, and eight to postdoctoral scholars in engineering. Nine grants (31%) were awarded to women and 20 grants (69%) were awarded to men. This means that these grants were applied for and awarded to approximately the percentage of women that one might expect, with 31% of the travel grants awarded to women at a time when women were 26% of the postdoctoral population at Princeton.

The Dependent Childcare Travel Grant Program was an extension of a program begun with an earlier seed grant, and the data presented here include the outcomes from both grants. This program provided grants of up to $500 a year to postdoctoral fellows and graduate students in the natural sciences and engineering for expenses they incurred for the care of children under the age of 12 years while they attended academic conferences and similar career-building events. Dependent Childcare Travel Grants were awarded to nine postdoctoral researchers and seven graduate students in the natural sciences and engineering. Ten (62%) of these grants were awarded to women and six (38%) were awarded to men (at a time when 31% of the graduate students and 26% of the postdoctoral fellows in the natural sciences and engineering were women). The grants could be used to reimburse any expenses incurred for child care, including (but not limited to) any of the following: hiring a caretaker at home; hiring someone to travel to the person's home to serve as a caretaker; hiring child care at a meeting site; arranging for children to travel to a caretaker; or arranging for a caretaker to travel to the meeting site.

The initial announcement of both the Dependent Childcare Travel Program (at the time of the first grant) and the Spouse/Partner Travel Program (in the spring of 2008) received a very warm response from faculty, postdoctoral researchers, and graduate students. In both instances, the thoughtful approaches were devised to alleviate the special pressures experienced by postdoctoral fellows and graduate students who have families and were singled out for accolades.

In order to assess the impact of the Spouse/Partner Travel Grants Program on the lives of the recipients, the 22 recipients still at Princeton were surveyed. Responses were received from 17 (77%) of them. Two questions were asked: "Please describe the difference that this grant made in your personal and professional life, including any effect it may have had on the quality of your experience at Princeton and on your research productivity," and "Please describe any changes/improvements you would make in the postdoctoral spouse/partner travel grant program if we are able to continue it going forward, and the rationale for any changes/improvements you propose." What was most striking about the responses to the first question was the near unanimity with which the recipients linked the reduction in stress and increase in quality of life that the grant provided with an improvement in their ability to focus on their research and increase their productivity. The responses to the second question indicated that the structure and organization of this grant program generally worked effectively for the recipients.

Implementation Highlights

Implementation of the programs proceeded without difficulty. The process was different for the two programs. For the Postdoctoral Spouse/Partner Travel Grant Program, applicants first had to demonstrate their eligibility. Processing of each grant took considerable time as, in each instance, the status of the spouse/partner as a graduate student or postdoctoral scholar in the natural sciences or engineering at an institution at least 150 miles from Princeton had to be verified. (It actually required considerable time simply to design the guidelines and the application forms for these grants.) Once eligibility was established, the recipient could submit travel receipts of up to $1500 for reimbursement during the subsequent year. Application for the Dependent Childcare Travel Grants was simpler; individuals applied for these grants by writing to the Office of the Dean of the Faculty with information about the dependent who would need child care and the academic conference or other event that the applicant would be attending, along with a detailed budget of up to $500. The grants were awarded directly based on this information.

Publicizing these programs on campus was a critical aspect of its success. Bringing the programs to the attention of postdoctoral fellows was a particular concern because at Princeton, these individuals do not have a community to which they relate other than in the laboratory in which they are located. At the beginning of each academic year, in order to ensure that all postdoctoral scholars and graduate students knew about the programs and how to apply for them, three key steps were followed: (1) the dean of the faculty sent a memo to all postdoctoral fellows describing the Spouse/Partner Travel Program and the Dependent Childcare Travel Program and how to apply for funding under each of the two programs; (2) the dean also sent a memo to all faculty members, all department chairs and center/institute directors, and all academic department managers describing the two programs and urging them to encourage individuals in their departments, centers, and institutes to apply for these funds as appropriate; and (3) the associate dean of the Graduate School sent a memo to all graduate students describing the menu of family-friendly programs available to them, including a description of the Dependent Care Travel Program and how to apply for funding under it.

In addition, the programs available to postdoctoral researchers were described on the Dean of the Faculty's home page on the Princeton University Web site in a section entitled "Family Friendly Programs" and as numbered memos posted on the site.[58,59] The Dependent Care Travel Program was described in detail on the Web site of the Graduate School.[60]

Lessons Learned

The original estimate of the need for the Postdoctoral Spouse/Partner Travel Grants was much lower than the ultimate demand revealed. At the same time, the estimate of the need for the Dependent Childcare Travel Grants was considerably greater. Nonetheless, although all requests for the child care travel grants could be fulfilled during the grant period, funds were depleted before all requests could be met for the spouse/partner grant funds. Many of the recipients of the spouse/partner grants were international postdoctoral researchers. It is possible that the incidence of scientist and engineer spouses and partners living apart is higher among this group. The overall experience with the Postdoctoral Spouse/Partner Travel Grant Program reinforced the belief that postdoctoral scholars have particular needs that are different from those of graduate students and faculty and that contribute to the vulnerability experienced by many of these individuals, especially women, during this phase of their careers. Next steps going forward will be to talk with postdoctoral fellows at Princeton to find out what difficulties they are experiencing and to think systematically about what Princeton might provide to mitigate these issues. The spouse/partner grant program targeted one of these needs, but there are likely other needs not yet identified.

If the Spouse/Partner Travel Grant Program is reinstated in the future, one change would be made in advertising it. As described above, memos were sent from the Dean of the Faculty to all postdoctoral research associates and fellows at Princeton, informing them of who was eligible for a grant and where to find the application forms. Future plans would include also notifying individuals to whom Princeton is offering postdoctoral appointments about the existence of the program. In this case, faculty would be encouraged to insert a brief paragraph about the Spouse/Partner Travel Program in the letter offering the postdoctoral appointment. This service could be a powerful recruiting tool, but it might also encourage other universities to provide funding for spouse/partner travel during the postdoctoral period.

There was one surprise in program implementation. According to Princeton's Office of Finance and Treasury, these grants had to be processed as supplemental income. In other words, the grants were taxable. In order to provide the funding specified in the grant proposal and the program material, grants had to include the money to pay for both the items for which the grant was awarded and the taxes on the amount granted. This situation resulted in the awarding of fewer grants than originally anticipated. Funding for the Dependent Childcare Travel Grant Program was not affected, as the institution was able to fulfill all the requests received, but it did affect the Postdoctoral Spouse/Partner Travel Grant Program in that there were insufficient funds to fulfill all the requests.

Sustainability

As originally planned, the program would have transitioned from being grant supported to being institution supported once the grant period concluded, especially because Princeton was committed from the start to supplementing the grant funds such that the programs could be made available to all postdoctoral researchers and graduate students. However, like other academic institutions facing the recent economic climate, Princeton had to reduce its support for a range of existing programs and has not been able to support new ones.

Nevertheless, the goal is to once again implement the Dependent Childcare Travel Awards, as these awards complement a similar program that Princeton has offered its faculty for almost a decade. Princeton has instituted a wide range of family-friendly policies and programs to help those who work and study at Princeton to balance their careers and family life. Those designed for faculty and for graduate students are posted on the institutional Web site.[61,62] Postdoctoral fellows and associates are supported by the work/life programs already available for all Princeton University employees.[63] Princeton employees are automatically eligible to participate in these programs, and those postdoctoral fellows who are not Princeton employees can become eligible to participate as well. At the same time, all these individuals have special difficulties and particular needs that are not addressed by the existing programs.

Conclusions

Both programs successfully provided targeted resources that alleviated particular stresses in the family lives of postdoctoral fellows and graduate students. Because stresses in family life frequently make it more difficult for individuals to perform at their highest capacity in their professional lives, it appears that these programs improved both the morale and productivity of the postdocs and graduate students who received awards through these initiatives. This view was supported by the responses received during the survey of those who received spouse/partner travel grants. Additional support was also gained for the view that the postdoctoral phase of an academic career—a phase experienced by almost all PhDs in the natural sciences and engineering—brings with it some unique stresses that are not present either during graduate school or once an individual has taken up a faculty (or other) appointment. Because there is substantial attrition from the faculty career track during the postdoctoral period—especially by women—more attention should be paid to the stresses endemic to this phase and to developing policies and programs that could help alleviate them.

CASE STUDY 12. TRANSITIONAL SUPPORT PROGRAM

Implementing organization: University of Rhode Island, Kingston, Rhode Island, USA (2007 Elsevier Foundation New Scholars Grant Awardee.)
Project leaders: Barbara Silver, PhD, and Helen Mederer, PhD.

Rationale and Goals

The Transitional Support Program challenged traditional mainstream tendencies to render invisible the differential impact caregiving challenges can have on women scientists' career advancement. It aimed to legitimize the need for flexible work arrangements for those whose careers are unfairly limited by these constraints, and to acknowledge formally the intersection of work and family in today's workplace, particularly for women in STEM. Specifically, it addressed the cultural contradiction surrounding breast-feeding in the workplace. That is, while new mothers experience strong societal encouragement to breast-feed and are increasingly returning to work soon after giving birth for economic and/or professional reasons, they often return to a workplace that lacks formal and informal support for breast-feeding or expressing milk. This program enabled the University of Rhode Island to launch a lactation program for student, staff, and faculty new mothers returning to work, to educate the wider university community about work/life issues, and to make connections and disseminate materials on the topic regionally.

The program goals were to (1) implement a lactation program at the University of Rhode Island; (2) develop a general program model for colleges and universities; (3) widely disseminate the lactation program model; (4) develop a work/life regional consortium; (5) provide support services to new mothers, particularly junior women in STEM; (6) win the Rhode Island "Breastfeeding Friendly Workplace" Gold award; and (7) collect institutional data.

Project Description and Outcomes

When faculty members depart the workplace for family leave purposes and then return, the workplace culture remains fundamentally untouched. This program sought to change that culture by offering work/life support while faculty are still on the job, over and above allowing parents to be off the job to meet family obligations. As such, this program provided ongoing services to junior women STEM caregivers to supplement the limited Parental Leave Policy that offers support at the birth or adoption of a child. The 3-year program consisted of two connected initiatives. The primary initiative sought to create a lactation policy and program for new breast-feeding mothers returning to the workplace. The second initiative was an education and awareness program designed to better educate the wider university community about work/life issues in general.

The program leaders went through formal channels to create a University Lactation Policy and to distribute guidelines for users and supervisors.[64] In addition, they contracted with a lactation consultant, who was available upon request to new mothers. They also established a lending resource library located in one secure lactation site and sponsored a brown-bag lunch series each semester that featured a variety of work/life topics and invited speakers from both inside and outside the university community. In the final year of the project, a model program plan was developed that included guidelines specific to colleges and universities: "College and University Lactation Programs: Some Additional Considerations".[65] This plan was disseminated to 50 regional colleges and universities in Rhode Island, Connecticut, and Massachusetts.

To foster efforts in building a regional consortium to establish workplace lactation programs, all eight higher education institutions in Rhode Island were contacted, as well as one school in Massachusetts. Each institutional visit included a representative of the Rhode Island Breastfeeding Coalition and led to the successful enrollment of four schools into the consortium. At least two of them are moving forward with their own lactation support services.

Many informational and outreach programs were initiated and events staged. For example, the university's work/life Web site was expanded to cover a wide range of work/life topics: family care, workplace flexibility, taking time off, health and wellness, professional development, financial planning and retirement, and culture and community. It now includes supplemental resource pages, such as supervisor resources, that deal with issues in the workplace and how to arrange a flexible schedule.[66] Two administrator breakfast workshops and one chairs' lunch workshop were offered, as well as a Work/Life Day 2009, which featured several events. A variety of small presentations at meetings were also held throughout the duration of the grant program. Work/life pamphlets and brochures were produced or revised and are now included in the university's New Employee Orientations. These documents have been distributed to the Human Resources and Affirmative Action offices, and are included in many Search Committee information packets. While brown-bag lunches were part of the program's support efforts for new mothers, they covered many other topics besides parenting, and were attended by a variety of employees, both men and women.

Implementation Highlights

Developing a formal breast-feeding policy approved by the university administration was a very positive and straightforward process, unlike many other work/life policy initiatives pursued in the past. The arguments favoring the policy included the need to conform to state breast-feeding laws, career advancement equity for women, transparency and consistency across different employee categories, and a better bottom line. The formal policy process required a public comment phase, which engendered a vigorously positive response from the campus community. Ultimately, the University of Rhode Island met the many criteria required by the Rhode Island Department of Health Breastfeeding Coalition and was the only Gold-level award recipient in 2009. This award afforded an opportunity to hold a campus awards ceremony and generated much publicity.

Three important educational events were held for university administrators. As noted, two breakfasts attracted an audience of 40–50 administrators each, and a combination of PowerPoint presentations and brainstorming sessions were used to increase awareness of work/life issues on campus. The Chairs' Lunch Workshop, featuring a similar format, highlighted issues that impact women as caregivers, particularly women in STEM fields.[67] Complementing these events were the many work/life brown-bag lunches and lunches for women in STEM.

The university's work/life Web site proved to be an important resource, as the Human Resources Office had not been particularly proactive in promoting a work/life agenda. The site includes not only information for employees, but also "how to" guidance for both supervisors and employees, along with general background on work/life issues.[68]

The construction of a work/life needs assessment, first developed for staff employees, is an ongoing initiative. The findings from this survey will be important in moving a work/life agenda forward at the university by providing data-driven support for policy improvements.[65] A similar survey for faculty will follow, and the reporting of staff results should encourage faculty participation. The intense marketing and promotion of this survey has placed work/life issues "on the radar" for many university employees for the first time, and solidifies the efforts of administrators over the past several years. Topic areas to be included in the assessment for various categories of employees include awareness of the availability of university work/life options; work/life needs; caregiving responsibilities (child and elder); dual-earner status; work/life conflict; level and sources of stress; job satisfaction; employee commitment; intention to leave; supervisory support; division of household labor; and division of daily activities.

Only mild interest exists for establishing an active regional network, most likely due to lack of active work/life initiatives at neighboring institutions. Although efforts to establish such a network have been concentrated mainly within the Human Resource department, at least two institutions were actively planning to pursue a lactation program. Gaining administrator buy-in for acquiring space for lactation sites has been a major concern. Space is a premium commodity at universities, so providing lactation space is not a priority unless interested parties advocate vigorously. Human-resources offices often operate within a traditional mind-set, so most work/life efforts have had to be encouraged by "outsiders" and active volunteer efforts. These obstacles can be overcome, but often require creativity and persistence.

Lessons Learned

As lactation spaces are not monitored other than by volunteers, it is difficult to collect robust data on use of these facilities. One positive result has been that, through active marketing and publicity, the university's Work/Life Committee has become fairly high profile and is now recognized by most employees as a fixed, permanent resource. Women in particular very much appreciate that an advocate exists on campus who is willing to champion work/life initiatives. Focusing on issues that are particularly resonant with men (such as elder care, dual careers, retirement options, and job flexibility) also has helped counter the perception that work/life balance is only a woman's issue. Continuous maintenance of high visibility will be important in mainstreaming a work/life agenda.

Promoting the business case for attention to work/life issues will be essential in promoting buy-in from administrators. While many, if not most, administrators feel they are well educated about what work/life balance or integration means, in reality they tend to have a one-dimensional view of workplace flexibility, believing it means simply providing paid leave or flexible schedules. In addition, many share the standard misperceptions about the cost/benefit of promoting a work-life agenda. Continuing proactive education, including providing local institutional examples of and anecdotes about the benefits of work/life programs, will be essential in moving traditional institutions forward.

Sustainability

In addition to establishing the university's award-winning lactation program, lactation policy, lactation facilities, and work/life Web site, this project has significantly increased awareness among employees and, perhaps more importantly, supervisors and administrators, about the importance of work/life supports and workplace flexibility for all employees. These benefits are especially important for caregivers, the majority of whom are women. All these features are now embedded at the university. A part-time work/life position in Human Resources has been approved, but has not been filled due to funding issues. However, having the approval bodes well for additional institutionalization of a work/life agenda in the future.

Through the many publications, brown-bag lunches, and workshops held during the project period, the significance of the efforts of the Work/Life Committee has been more fully recognized and the members of the committee are now known and endorsed across campus as institutional advocates. The development of a Work/Life Needs Assessment may be the most important legacy of this project. The findings will be revealing and compelling for university supervisors and administrators and should provide the vehicle through which more change can occur.

In addition to these internal advances, the development of a program model for colleges and universities, regional outreach, and the establishment of a relationship with the Rhode Island Department of Health and other area schools have all laid the groundwork for future collaborations.

Conclusions

The University of Rhode Island launched an award-winning lactation program for student, staff, and faculty new mothers returning to work or school and developed a program model to share with other institutions. In addition, greater awareness of work/life issues was created throughout the university via lunches, educational workshops, a comprehensive work/life Web site, and literature dissemination.

PRACTICAL TOOLS

Advocacy Letter to Professional Societies

(Developed by the University of Massachusetts-Amherst STEM Family Travel Initiative.)

Dear (conference/workshop organizer):

As an attendee of your meeting (and member of your society), I am writing to ask for your support in making this event as attainable as possible for young women and dual-career couples who are often limited by dependent care restraints.

A recent survey showed that professional travel for faculty (primarily women) who provide the primary dependent care within a family remains a constant professional hurdle for those who seek tenure in science, technology, engineering, and mathematics disciplines. It remains a challenge to midcareer women faculty and other women who wish to remain competitive throughout their careers. The cost of child care at a meeting runs at $150–250/day using a professional nanny. The additional cost of bringing a child to a meeting varies with the price of airline tickets but runs on the order of $500 or more. Some children require that a familiar caregiver travel with them, while others are comfortable with new on-site providers. These expenses are generally not reimbursable on faculty grants due to restrictions on federal and state funding.

Quite often we find that conference organizers and even small professional societies with an interest in promoting women are unsure how to help. The arrangement of on-site child care, most appropriate for large organizations (and implemented regularly, for instance, by the ACS) may not be appropriate for smaller groups. Other ideas you may wish to consider in the future include

- Developing a list of available, reliable providers near the conference.
- Providing modest financial support for child care to attendees demonstrating need.
- Arranging an electronic bulletin board for attendees of your conference who may be willing to split the costs of a professional nanny.
- Making sure that children are welcome and safe in the public areas/eating rooms surrounding the conference itself.
- Providing comfortable nursing stations for new mothers.

I hope this letter has served to make you aware of the issues facing women scientists traveling for professional reasons.

Sincerely,
Dr Professor Female Traveler

Strategic Steps for Effective Implementation of Family-Friendly Policies

(Adapted from the approach taken by the University of Rhode Island Transitional Support Program to foster the creation of on-campus lactation facilities.)

- Understand the formal procedural steps your institution uses to establish policy. Introduce the idea to the appropriate people.
- Identify influential individuals and/or groups on campus who are supportive of the initiative to coauthor or otherwise support the policy request.
- Carefully select the author of the request, especially if resistance is expected. Your human resources department may or may not be the most effective source, depending on the institution. Women's commissions, equity councils, diversity officers, etc., may be more successful. A work/life director or office is obviously another source.
- Develop a rationale, or case statement, referring to state law, the business case, examples of peer institutions' programs, and the projected need at your institution.
- Utilize the larger agenda of work/life balance, workplace flexibility, equity, and diversity to frame your request. The rationale for promoting workplace flexibility is readily available from many sources.
- Frame support of the initiative as a workplace and workforce issue, rather than as a women's issue. Today there are as many women in the workforce as men, and dual-earner households are the norm. Supporting family-friendly initiatives is supporting the next generation of workers; it is not simply an accommodation for women.
- Develop a policy statement and set of guidelines.
- If the policy approval process includes a public comment period, take advantage of this requirement by encouraging your networks to respond. Comments will likely be overwhelmingly positive. Track comments and use them to your advantage.
- Have a management plan, including a timeline; identify a person who will be responsible for promoting the program, collecting data, and overseeing facilities.
- Have a marketing plan, including literature, Web sites, brown-bag lunches, announcements, and visits to departmental meetings, the Deans' Council, etc. Consider making it part of a work/life Web site.

Assessing Child Care Needs for Members of Professional Societies at Meetings

(Developed by the University of Massachusetts-Amherst STEM Family Travel Initiative.)

Some professional societies offer on-site day care at their conference facilities using a professional provider. STEM FTI would like to see more such facilities at conferences if they are likely to be popular.

Use this form to tell us your level of interest in having on-site child care available at a conference site (using an insured provider hired by the professional society organizing the event).

We are seeking statistical information to submit to professional societies in an effort to make the case for the utility of child care services to their members. Your specific personal information will not be forwarded beyond STEM FTI. Please include your name and e-mail so that we may contact you with questions and avoid duplicate submissions.

Name (required)

E-mail address (required)

Primary affiliation

Department

Institution/organization

Your position: faculty, administrator, scientist, postdoc, student

Number of children of day care age (up to 16 years old) or potentially using care

Name of professional society

(Select one from the list or choose "Other" and type in name)

American Institute of Chemical Engineers

American Physical Society

Materials Research Society

Other

Are you a regular dues-paying member of this society? yes | no

How many national or "main" meetings for this particular society have you attended in the past 5 years?

Has having children curtailed your attendance at this society's meetings within the past 5 years? yes | no

Have child care issues curtailed your participation in this professional society other than in terms of attendance (for example, have you attended the meeting but not been able to attend certain sessions or business meetings that you otherwise would have)? yes | no

Have child care issues impacted your ability to volunteer in this professional society? For example, to chair/organize sessions or symposia or participate more fully in the society's leadership? yes | no

I would use on-site professional child care if it were free yes | no

I would use on-site professional child care even if I had to pay for it yes | no

If child care were available at the meeting sites, I would likely (greater than 50% chance) attend conferences organized by this society in 2012 | 2013 | 2014 | 2015

If child care were not available, I would be less likely to attend future meetings true | false

PART 3

Advancing Comprehensive Solutions

Mentoring and Networking

Research is not for the faint of heart. I am always under stress—to write more, review it faster, get more grants, all the while being a perfect mentor and good leader in the department. If I didn't love it, it would not be worth it. **—A woman working in the biological sciences, age 46–55 years, divorced, USA**

I have a team of researchers at different levels who are able to perform all types of tasks. **—A woman working in neuroscience, age 36–45 years, married/ partnered, Australia**

As much of this book illustrates, the cultures and policies of scientific workplaces exert a strong influence on the individuals who work in them and on their perceptions of work/life issues. These workplaces can support the career growth and development of those whom they employ and/or educate by becoming aware of and supporting effective mentoring and networking, particularly in light of balancing professional responsibilities with personal priorities. Mentors can be superb models of meeting the challenges of fulfilling the multiple roles of a science, technology, engineering, and mathematics (STEM) professional, family member, and community member. Mentors can also articulate vital perspectives on how to pursue a successful career while also devoting important time and effort to life away from work. Networking with others who may face similar challenges can also be extremely useful in identifying solutions that may work for particular circumstances.

In this chapter, concepts are presented in the context of strategies that individuals can deploy in their own career decision making. A useful framework is to consider these strategies as five tools in a career toolbox that can be used when needed, either singly or in combination. The five concepts—self-analysis, mentoring, networking, coaching, and sponsoring—are described and discussed below in the second person to more effectively convey their utility. Perspectives and specific action items on mentoring as it relates to those in the STEM fields have been covered in depth by one of the authors in a recently published book.[69]

SELF-ANALYSIS

As a first step, and as a continuous process, introspection is pivotal to an individual's understanding his or her career goals and aspirations. The essential element is to cultivate an awareness of what motivates you in both your work and "away from work" lives. These motivations do vary widely from individual to individual and over time as careers develop, mature, reach a plateau, or encounter obstacles. Some useful points to reflect upon at any time may include (1) What are my most critical career concerns right now? (2) What are my most critical life concerns right now? (3) What is my ideal job? and (4) What are the new skills or abilities that I think I need?

Self-understanding is obviously a highly individualistic and personal undertaking. It is difficult to articulate a specific approach that may work for everyone. For some people, acquiring their desired level of self-knowledge may be a long and painful process, while others may find it relatively easy and straightforward. A part of thinking through these issues is to ponder what constitute your own personal priorities, values, interests, and aptitudes. Another aspect is considering how your career meshes with your personal life and any disconnections that you perceive between what you currently have and what you aspire to. Knowing and understanding the communities with which you feel the strongest affiliations are essential, whether they are your cultural community of origin, specific geographic settings, or workplace and disciplinary environments. Sometimes the other tools in the toolkit, presented below, can also be useful in your journey of discovery toward understanding of yourself. It is important to remember than no one person has a perfect career or a perfect life, despite how it may appear.

MENTORING

Today there are likely as many perspectives on mentoring as there are books on the topic. However, there are differences in the way we define "mentors", "advisors", "coaches", "sponsors", and "supervisors". Here, a mentor is a wise and trusted person who guides, protects, and promotes the protégé's (or mentee's) career. An advisor is someone who offers advice from a perspective of wisdom or authority. A coach helps one develop specific skills and abilities, often on a fee basis. A sponsor advocates and provides tactical support for one's advancement. A supervisor ("boss") has the official task of overseeing one's work. For those who are still in training or early career-development phases, it is important to understand that a mentor is not, by definition, the PhD advisor or postdoctoral supervisor. But many graduate and postdoctoral advisors and supervisors are mentors in the best sense of the term. As well, some individuals may serve several of these roles as you seek the best mentoring for yourself.

Identifying the best mentors to suit your needs at a particular time is a highly individualized undertaking, but certain steps can enhance the likelihood that you will seek and find the perspectives that you need. Being prepared for potential mentoring experiences is built on a foundation of self-reflection, as noted above. This involves first identifying the key areas in which you need mentoring. For some people, enhancing skills and abilities in public speaking, scientific writing, or priority setting may be an area of need. For others, assessing the best workplace in which to pursue professional interests would be uppermost. Appropriate mentors can also help with resolving work/life issues, life-partner issues, or adapting to unfamiliar cultures or places. The second step is to focus on the critical concerns of your current career stage. These relative priorities will change as you move through a career, but good mentoring can help you to concentrate on the most important of these priorities at appropriate times. Third, once you start a relationship with your mentors, it is important from the first stages to develop action steps that keep your mentoring goals on track. These steps can include the mutual setting of outcomes to achieve during the mentoring relationship; formulating guidelines for how you would like to proceed (including mode of interaction and topics that may be "off limits" during the mentoring experience); and agreeing upon a regular meeting or contact schedule. Once these parameters are set, both mentor and protégé will want to ensure they adhere to the agenda and schedule; give and receive positive feedback; review outcomes and accomplishments on a consistent basis; ask questions and be an excellent listener; and seek out new resources and opportunities that can enhance the overall mentoring experience. A fourth area encompasses recognizing the "do's and don'ts" of mentoring relationships. In brief, these rules include being ethical and straightforward by presenting yourself honestly and thoughtfully; having a sense of humor; not putting your mentor in an awkward position; realizing that your actions (good or bad) will often have larger consequences; and seeking the information and advice that you need. A fifth and final step is to recognize that your mentors are not miracle workers; you have to make things happen for yourself by being honest, confronting painful realities forthrightly, and moving forward rather than attempting to redesign or relive past mistakes.

It is very reasonable to expect your mentors to help you identify the balance between personal fulfillment and professional success that is right for you, to question you on the level of satisfaction you feel with the choices you are making, to understand your current situation and the systems in which you live and work, and to help you recognize your strengths and weaknesses. No one individual is likely to be able to do all of the above for you. Therefore, you should keep in mind the concept of a "panel" or "board" of mentors—i.e., a group of individuals who, in the aggregate, can provide the perspective and guidance you seek.

NETWORKING

This third tool in the career toolkit is a strong complement to mentoring. Networking is more than just getting to know others in your field or work sector. It is a career-long endeavor that can provide information not only for your own career decisions, but also for learning about matters that might be relevant to the content of your work. Networking occurs in any arena where people might find common ground—professional meetings, the workplace, community and social events, in volunteer work settings with professional and community organizations—and through a variety of social and career-related media (e.g., LinkedIn, Web sites, and professional society affinity groups). If you are of introverted temperament (and many STEM professionals are), one of the most terrifying situations can be entering a room where you know few, if any, of the persons there. However, it is amazing how easy it is to start conversations if you merely ask how people got started in their chosen profession or, in a nonwork context, how they got involved with a community organization. That question can often lead to discussions on what individuals may like about their particular field and the advantages and disadvantages of their chosen career pathway. Such discussions can complement your own ongoing process of introspection and making career decisions.

Some of the concepts that apply to mentoring can be applicable in the networking context as well, as mentoring opportunities can arise from networking encounters. For individuals at the same career stage or level, peer-to-peer mentoring activities can result from networking activities, and vice versa. Often this type of networking can assist with consideration of points such as "Is it time for me to 'move on'? Have I developed the skill sets that I need? Am I focusing my efforts in the most productive manner and directions? Do I know what I need to be doing in preparation for my next career phase?" Such peers will likely have transitional goals similar to yours, and can provide positive reinforcement for the changes you are contemplating and support in helping you let go of what you feel you "should" do or want.

Networking can also be beneficial as you ponder crucial questions on your career's path: "What must I stop doing?", "What must I start doing?", and "What must I continue doing?" Anyone who has moved from a full-time bench research position into a supervisory role (whether as an industry manager or a faculty member, for example) quickly discovers that new tasks arise and that others must now be delegated to colleagues. Here, perspectives from peers and potential mentors are extremely helpful, whether one is pondering a career change or grappling with being overwhelmed in a current position.

Effective networking does demand a degree of proactivity, as "lucky breaks" cannot be counted on to occur when you need them. You cannot assume that you will "bump into" the right person at the right time with the right opportunity. Enhancing your efforts in networking is essential for connecting with people who can point you in the right direction and who can refer you to others. The more the people with whom you establish connections, the more likely you are to acquire the information or contacts that you need.

COACHING

As noted in the introductory section of this chapter, the definition of a coach is someone who helps you with specific skill and ability development, often on a fee basis. In a broader context, most people are familiar with the term "coach" as it relates to organized sports, but there are now many individuals who work in this area, serving as life coaches, executive coaches, business coaches, and career coaches. In most cases, these types of personal or professional coaches do not have direct experience in one's own field (unlike in most mentoring relationships among persons in STEM). The concept of coaching has, however, gained increased stature among STEM professionals over the past decade, although professionals in many other fields have a longer history of experience with career coaches. Some organizations, particularly within industry, provide coaching for employees with technical backgrounds so that they can become more effective supervisors and leaders. To date, such leadership coaching has not been widely deployed in academia, but some professional societies in

STEM are beginning to recognize its importance for the career advancement of their members.

For the STEM professional, the decision to employ a coach may result from the desire to improve performance on the current job or to develop skills that would enhance opportunities for advancement. Executive management skills, interpersonal communication skills, or even time management skills are examples of areas in which coaches can work with STEM clients. When such coaches are employed, there is usually a defined and measurable goal targeted to the client's specific needs. Therefore, it is essential to first determine exactly what your needs are and to ensure that your chosen coach can provide the type and extent of services required.

SPONSORING

If the concept of career coaching has been late in coming to the world of STEM, sponsoring is an even less well-known concept. As noted, a sponsor advocates and provides tactical support for your advancement, often in the organization where you are employed. In general, such an individual goes well beyond such roles as mentor and networking colleague in order to make a strong case for your suitability for employment and match to the organization. Elements of sponsorship have long been a part of academic advancement in science fields, particularly in those instances where well-known scientists leveraged their reputations and influence to secure good positions for their graduate students or postdoctoral fellows. However, the narrow concept of promoting one's own students is a much less effective pathway to success for the vast majority of individuals, due to both the dynamics of today's job marketplace and a greater sensitivity to achieving fairness and equity. Today, the best sponsors can demystify organizational processes and cultures for you, are cognizant of what it takes to advance in the organization, and can assess your fit for particular professional pathways. They are willing to stake their reputation to support your advancement and be an advocate for you because they have confidence in your abilities and anticipated success. If you are sponsored in such manner, you do bear the pressure of expectations to fulfill the potential that your sponsor perceived.

SOME CONCLUDING THOUGHTS

The principles of mentoring, networking, coaching, and sponsoring are powerful when implementation strategies for each process are well thought out and tactically deployed at both the individual and institutional levels. Coupled with self-awareness and introspection, these types of relationships allow individuals to secure their career growth and development by (1) acquiring the appropriate professional credentials; (2) learning to recognize professional opportunities; (3) recovering from and rectifying mistakes and missteps; (4) dealing with their own biases and misconceptions; (5) creating opportunities for others; (6) knowing when to move on; and (7) stretching beyond normal comfort zones in taking strategic risks. In turn, organizations and institutions can facilitate resolution of career transitions and challenges that their employees and future employees face by acknowledging that each person represents a concatenation of personal life priorities, career priorities, and interests in the community at large.

Implicit Bias and the Workplace

I am concerned that saying no to service work will negatively impact my career.
—**A man working in biological sciences, age 26–35 years, single, Canada**

In my institution, there is little opportunity to go up in rank based on scientific merit alone. —**A man working in electrical engineering, age 36–45 years, married/partnered, Netherlands**

Underlying many of the struggles women in science, technology, engineering, and mathematics (STEM) endure, in both advancing their careers and finding time and energy for family life, is the issue of implicit bias. Implicit bias is also the "elephant in the room" that will have to be shoved aside if promising programs such as those described in the case studies are ever to succeed fully. Granted, prejudice exists throughout human culture. The body of literature committed to understanding why this seemingly negative quality has persisted through our evolution into modern times is expansive. What we do know is that we are social creatures, and recognizing that there is an "us" and a "them" probably conferred serious historic advantages. The problem is that this response, although it perhaps served a function when we were transitioning from nomadic tribes to agrarian societies, has become a hindrance to corporate and academic progress. When we make decisions based on ideas of what "us" means, we often do so informed by the culture in which we were raised and with a strong emotional basis rather than a logical one. Unfortunately, while this tendency is pervasive, scientists and engineers often think that they have evolved beyond the rest of human society and are thus immune to allowing such passion to influence their judgment. However, studies demonstrate this is not the case.

Recognizing that our prejudices occur not only at a conscious level but also an unconscious one is important for understanding how to inoculate against them. While we may think we are focusing on one immediate thing, our brain is busy making other judgments and decisions about other aspects of that thing. These assessments are based on the memories and emotions that inform our perspective. This phenomenon is best demonstrated by a video that asks the viewer to count the number of times a ball is passed between players in white shirts. While the action occurs, other people in black shirts elsewhere onscreen are passing a different ball. Midway through the exercise, a man in a gorilla suit walks between the players, beats his chest, and then walks off screen. In a classic demonstration of selective attention, although everyone who watches the video of course sees the man in the gorilla suit when he appears, many viewers completely fail to notice him.

As this anecdote illustrates, oftentimes, the world as we perceive it may not be the world as it actually is. A different video that made the rounds on the Internet a few years ago explained that the amount of information with which we are inundated daily, monthly, and yearly has been increasing at an exponential rate. Some studies estimate that at any given moment, we are exposed on average to 11 million different things in our environment; however, our brain permits us to process only about 50 things at a time. As a consequence, there is a tremendous risk that we will miss things that do not fit into our limited view based on our cognitive processing capacity. Part of how our brain copes with this limitation is by injunctification.[70] Injunctification posits that we are motivated to deem the current state of things we see as natural and desirable, leading to the defense of the status quo. Thus, for example, people are likely to defend the idea that women do not like math or engineering because they are not well represented in the field; they consider this supposed discomfort to be the reason women do not pursue these professions, rather than considering that there may be other barriers to women's participation. That perception is a very serious problem.

One argument against the status quo is that countries with less progressive cultures have more women going into STEM professions than is currently seen in the United States. Women in many countries in the Middle East and Central Asia are earning degrees in STEM fields at unprecedented rates (although some cultures are not so progressive that women are free to practice their profession once they have earned a degree). Understanding the manner in which culture influences the decisions we make, the activities we pursue, and the beliefs we hold is important to combating these influences. Certain ideas are associated with certain values, a message that is consistently reinforced in our culture, whether it is in regard to appearances, constructed gender roles, racial associations, sexual preferences, or religious beliefs. Our interests in engineering a better scientific workplace and implementing successful strategies is overcoming the notion that "only men do science".

A classic study asked high school students to draw a scientist. With great consistency, the students depicted a white man in a laboratory coat with glasses.[71] This stereotypical response alone is a problem. An even bigger problem is that when scientists were asked to participate in the same exercise, they tended to produce the same images as the high school students. This association—that scientists are men—is reinforced continually throughout the media, academia, and popular culture. To examine one's own biases, the Implicit Association Test (IAT), developed by researchers at Harvard, allows one to test one's own preconceptions based on how quickly one responds to various word pairings.[72] Although not without its critics and shortcomings, the IAT is still informative and a great jumping-off point for exploring the impact subtle cultural cues have on our personal development.

Understanding these biases and associations is also important because they have a chilling effect not just on efforts to recruit girls into science and engineering, but also on perceptions of women in these fields. These subtle associations manifest in big ways. For example, stereotype threat is the fear of performing poorly in a particular field where our gender or race is believed to be inferior, thus reinforcing the stereotype.[73] Researchers who study stereotype threat have demonstrated that girls as young as 9 years start to internalize the message that "math is hard" and that it is probably something at which boys are better. Although these associations begin at a young age, they persist in our subconscious and ultimately have an impact on decisions regarding hiring, promotion, and recognition. The ensuing implications are dire for the retention of women in STEM fields as well as in other parts of the workforce. The remainder of this chapter summarizes studies from a variety of fields and describes a project that applies many of the principles gleaned from these studies. The chapter concludes with a list of best practices for minimizing the impact of subconscious bias.

WHAT'S IN A SCIENTIST'S NAME?

As mentioned above, scientists may be particularly loath to concede that they, too, are influenced by the culture in which they were raised. Most presumably would espouse an egalitarian worldview that does not endorse an innate difference between genders in their ability to perform high-quality research. However, beliefs do not seem to translate into unbiased evaluation of individuals, suggesting that a conscious worldview is not always sufficient to overcome implicit biases. Perhaps it is less surprising that only a handful of studies have examined the impact of unconscious bias upon hiring decisions in academia.

One of the approaches frequently used in sociological research in this area is to take a standard measure of evaluation—a resume or curriculum vitae (CV), for example—and then change one facet, such as the gender or race of the individual to whom it belongs. The CVs or resumes, identical save for that single variable, are then handed out to individuals qualified to evaluate the professional criteria. In one study, a CV for a psychology professor position was being evaluated by primary investigators in the field. In a second study, an application package for a laboratory manager position was assessed. The only variable that differed in each of these two studies was whether the individual being evaluated had a man's or a woman's fictitious name at the top of the CV.

In both instances, the "female" candidate fared worse than the male candidate by a significant margin. Perhaps more importantly, the quality of the female applicant's resume was undervalued by both the men and women doing the evaluation, demonstrating that it is not just men who are biased against women in science. In the case of the psychology professor position, the study revealed that the evaluators more positively valued the man's research, teaching, and service background; further, it confirmed previous data indicating that search committees are more likely to hire a man at the associate professor level—although a woman is typically deemed better suited toward an assistant professorship.[74] In the application package for the laboratory manager position, the individual being evaluated was a recent graduate with a bachelor's degree and some prior research experience.[75] The "female" applying for that position was viewed as less worthy of mentoring, less competent, less desirable as a new hire, and was offered less financial compensation. These results are distressing, particularly the fact that the hypothetical search committee of psychologists would demonstrate such partiality, given that there is a substantial likelihood that they would be routinely exposed to papers regarding the topic of implicit bias during their training and in the course of their work.

While the data in these studies would seem difficult to refute, there are those who try to minimize the significance of such results. Undoubtedly most of the study participants would deny being consciously biased against women in science. However, Ben Barres, a noted neuroscientist, has written eloquently on this subject based on his firsthand experience with gender bias and double standards, having formerly been known as Barbara Barres. In perhaps the single most telling anecdote, he recounts how, after a highly successful presentation at the institution where he earned his PhD, a friend told him that after the applause died down he heard one professor remarking to another, "Ben Barres's work is much better than his sister's". In fact, he was actually just recalling the same scientist's presentation from a few years earlier.[76] The conclusion that can be drawn from these studies is that scientists are just as biased as the rest of humanity. Acknowledging this reality is crucial if we are to move forward, and it should not be permitted to interfere with evaluations that should be based on scholarly merit rather than gender.

BLIND ORCHESTRAL AUDITIONS

Orchestras, like the fields of science and engineering, have historically had a low representation of women in their ranks. In part, this is because many music directors, who have historically had a significant influence over hiring, had vocally expressed the opinion that, based on auditions, women were less talented musicians than men. The traditional progression for the musically elite (man) was to train with the best (men) and then be recommended for auditions with the top-tier orchestras. Social trends in the 1970s, along with many other aspects of the culture, were moving toward a more democratic system, one based less on grooming and social nepotism and more on pure ability. As a consequence, a substantially greater number of individuals were auditioning for orchestras because openings and auditions were announced more broadly. In a further effort to ensure an unbiased audition process, it became routine for the individual performing to be placed behind a screen so that nothing about that individual except the performance was being evaluated. This intervention is presumably one reason the number of female musicians in symphonies began to increase.

However, not all musical groups opted to use the screen. Using data from auditions and hiring numbers, Claudia Goldin and Cecelia Rouse compared the numbers of women hired in orchestras that used a screen compared with those that did not between 1950 and 1995.[77] These data allowed the researchers to determine whether bias played a role in the number of women hired by eight separate orchestras. Although broadening the number of opportunities to audition increased the representation of women on its own, the use of a screen increased the likelihood that a woman would be hired by roughly one-third. The data from this study demonstrate that whenever it is possible, masking the identity of the individual being evaluated to focus specifically on the performance quality being evaluated is the best policy. Additionally, the more broadly disseminated the solicitations are for a position, the greater the chance of getting the best quality applicants.

DOUBLE-BLIND LITERATURE REVIEWS

Many scientific journals perform a double-blind peer review of submitted literature, a system of evaluation in which neither the author's nor the reviewer's identity is revealed to the other. The double-blind system is not without its critics (the small populations in certain fields sometimes mean that the primary investigator may be guessed from the subject matter, and the process adds to the administrative burden on the publisher's side). However, the system is superior to single-blind review in terms of combating gender bias related to authorship.

A certain ecology journal transitioned from single-blind review to double blind in 2001. Using this opportunity to compare the rate of publication by each gender before and after the transition for several years on either side of change, A.E. Budden et al. initiated a study to investigate the outcomes of this transition.[78] After analyzing the numbers, as well as comparing them with representation of female authors in other major ecology publications, they found that the double-blind review process led to a nearly 8% increase in the number of articles published by women relative to the total number in just a few years. Eight percent may not sound like a substantial increase, but women are poorly represented in the upper echelons of the ecology field, so that increase may have a larger trickle-down effect. Furthermore, if the double-blind review increases the equity of the journal review process by reducing the opportunity for bias and subsequently leading to an increase in the number of women publishing, removing one obstacle from women's ability to succeed is a step in the right direction. A substantial number of publications are necessary for competitive positioning when applying for faculty positions and getting tenure, as well as for winning scholarly awards; therefore, it is only logical that all disciplines should adopt processes that reduce bias and thus permit evaluators to focus exclusively on the quality of the science.

SUCCESS AND LIKEABILITY DO NOT GO HAND IN HAND (FOR WOMEN)

Heidi Roizen is a highly successful, award-winning executive, venture capitalist, and entrepreneur. Her resume demonstrates her talents in a range of areas as well as her ability to adroitly recognize and fluidly take on challenging new tasks while climbing the corporate ladder. Stanford Professor Frank Flynn, PhD, developed an experiment using Roizen's stellar resume as the framework to construct a case study to examine attitudes toward success and likeability as they relate to gender. Half of the students in a Harvard Business School class received a case with her name included in a document delineating her career achievements; the other half received the same case except that "Heidi" Roizen was changed to "Howard" Roizen throughout the document.[79] Students were then asked to read through the resume and evaluate the "candidate" for various qualities.

While analysis showed that students found Heidi/Howard to be equally competent, they were much more severe in judging Heidi's personality. They did not like her and generally did not want to hire or work with her. They were put off by her aggressive nature and found her "selfish". The same cannot be said for their evaluations of "Howard". This result is consistent with other literature, which generally finds that success negatively correlates with likeability for women. This equation is borne out in the real world when employees are interviewed by the press; regardless of whether the workplace is the New York publishing world or a Silicon Valley tech start-up, high-achieving women are consistently represented as odious and demanding. This negative association between women and success is a constant struggle to women's advancement and accounts at least partly for the lack of female leadership at technology and pharmaceutical companies, medical schools, and Fortune 500 corporations. The one upside to the above findings is that the negative correlation between likeability and success can be reduced when high-achieving women develop personal relationships with their colleagues and others; research shows that men tend to judge accomplished women they know beyond a one-dimensional context less harshly. However, such familiarity still does not eradicate the problem.

THE SELECTIVE ABSENCE OF FEMALE CONFERENCE SPEAKERS

Conferences are an important opportunity for individuals to present their research, disseminate their findings, receive feedback on their results, initiate collaborations, and network with other experts in their field. Yet women tend to be heavily underrepresented among invited speakers at disciplinary conferences. The reasons for this are complex and multifaceted. There is, of course, variation among disciplines in their representation of women. One recent study showed that the likelihood of women being invited to speak depends on the representation of women and men on conference organizing committees. In several subdisciplines of primatology, for example, women have comprised more than half the field for the last few decades. However, when the study authors examined the number of invited female speakers who participated in symposia over the past two decades (separate from those who requested the opportunity to present their work), they found that the composition of the selection committee had a tremendous impact on the number of women speakers invited. All-female and mixed-composition committees invited women speakers at a rate commensurate with the representation of established leaders in the field. An all-male committee, on the other hand, invited 20–35% fewer women than would be expected as symposium speakers. The authors propose that the gender inequity seen with the all-male committee is due most likely to subconscious bias or homophily (the tendency to want to bond with one's own kind), a term that presumably comes up with some frequency in primatology.[80]

One aspect of this study that was not addressed concerned how many women were invited to speak compared with how many accepted the offers. Another recent study indicated that in some disciplines, although the number of women invited is representative of the populations within the discipline or hosting society, many women decline the opportunity to speak.[81] This reluctance could certainly be a very valid explanation for the low representation of women in conference symposia in the field being examined—evolutionary biology—a discipline in which women are significantly more poorly represented than in primatology. However, the reasons are perhaps more complicated than simply that women do not want to speak on the record. Women still face greater scrutiny online, during interviews, via applications, by review panels, and in all other aspects of their scientific careers due to implicit bias. So, although women might be turning down an opportunity to speak, thus declining the chance to promote their work and serve as a role model, at the end of the day the implicit bias that does not associate women with science—or rather, that associates science with men—may be a large part of the underlying source of the discrepancy. It would be interesting to see whether the invitation coming from an all-female versus all-male selection committee had any impact on the acceptance rate, and whether there is a tipping point for a representation level in a particular field that would increase the likelihood of more women accepting invitations.

The key lesson of both these studies is that bias may play a role in the representation of women at conferences, which is one more way that women wind up appearing marginalized in the STEM fields and thus publically presenting fewer positive role models and limiting their own career networks. In addition to actively encouraging greater participation by women at conferences, an approach designed to minimize implicit bias should include creating heterogeneous committees. Furthermore, assuring all participants have access to the financial and family-care accommodations necessary to attend conferences is a step in the right direction toward increasing the representation of women in symposia.

THE POWER OF LANGUAGE

Words have the power, subtly or overtly, to shape perspectives and color the accomplishments listed on a person's CV or resume. The tints used can impact dramatically how natural the final image appears. Coloring a picture of a zebra with green and purple stripes might make for an interesting image, but it is not a very realistic depiction. In the same manner, using a certain vocabulary to describe women and another set of words to describe men can shift how realistically one might view an individual's fit for a particular job. Many studies have demonstrated that when individuals are crafting letters of recommendation for women, they choose descriptive terms different from those they use for men.

When writing about women, individuals tend to focus on the candidate's ability to nurture, her dependability, her capacity as a team player, and perhaps her ability to balance her obligations as a mother as well as a scientist. They use words such as "conscientious", "methodical", and "dependable".[82] On the other hand, words used to describe men focus on their intellect and scientific achievements, including terms such as "brilliant", "analytical", "talented", and "results". Consequently, even though both of two letters might be very positive, each paints a very different picture of the candidate's relative ability to contribute to the institution—and thus, how he or she is viewed in terms of fit for a particular position.[83] As a consequence, considering the language being used when crafting a recommendation letter is very important. Using gender-neutral or even conventionally masculine terms, to describe a woman is advisable. T. Schmader has compiled a complete list of recommended terms.[82]

In addition to its impact upon letters of recommendation, certain language in a job description can bias a prospective hire. For example, a job advertisement that emphasizes company culture—e.g., a tech start-up that sounds more like a fraternity house than a workplace—is likely to "turn off" an applicant who is not interested in walking into an office that is borderline hostile to women. Along the same lines, when reading a solicitation for a particular award named after a pioneer in the field, someone considering candidates for that award might be swayed by the subconscious influence of the name of the award to nominate someone who seems to fit the standard to receive that accolade because he or she resembles the pioneer. Giving consideration to the language used in writing recommendation letters and in creating positions, endowments, and awards; and refraining from using names that indicate some particular example that no longer resembles the potential breadth and diversity of the STEM enterprise would be positive steps toward creating a more inclusive academic community that focuses on actual achievements, not stereotypes.

THE AWARDS PROJECT

Drawing on many of the principles outlined within this chapter, which emphasize focusing on achievement by increasing transparency and minimizing opportunities for bias, it may be instructive to review a project undertaken by the Association of Women in Science (AWIS) regarding recognition. Scholarly awards from disciplinary societies are an important benchmark of achievement in academic culture. They are used in evaluating candidates for hiring, tenure, and promotions. Workplace management studies have shown that people would rather be recognized for their achievements than given raises, and this finding is particularly salient in the academic environment, which does not attract people for the money as much as for the opportunity to make outstanding intellectual contributions to the body of scientific knowledge.

Anecdotally, it has been said that women were underrepresented among winners of scholarly awards given by disciplinary societies relative to the available pool of women holding positions in the upper echelons of academia and industry. The late Phoebe S. Leboy, PhD, a past AWIS president and professor at the University of Pennsylvania, examined a wide range of scientific societies and found this characterization to be accurate, as shown in Figure 8.21. Additionally, women were more likely to be society president than winners of a scholarly award. Furthermore, women were overrepresented among winners of mentoring and service awards relative to the expected pool, and women won particularly few scholarly awards when there were "women only" awards available.[84]

Recognizing that this disparity is a serious concern for the promotion and retention of women in STEM, AWIS sought and was awarded a grant to study ways to increase the transparency and equity of the awards process.[85] The resulting project, Advancing Ways of Awarding Recognition in Disciplinary Societies (AWARDS), supported a workshop in 2010 to which seven scientific societies representing a wide range of STEM disciplines[86] were invited. At the workshop, various aspects of the awards process were examined.

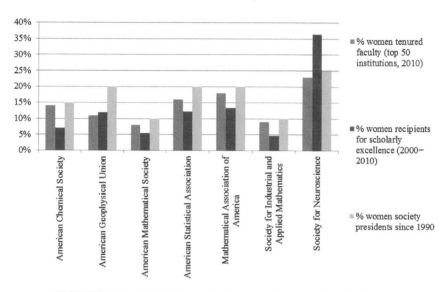

FIGURE 8.21   Scholarly awards to women by professional societies.

The recommendations to increase the transparency and thereby the equity of the awards process involved a wide range of approaches and topics. Central was the idea that implicit bias influences many different aspects of the process. Implicit bias training at the beginning of the workshop was central to the discussion; in this way, all participants were helped both to understand that everyone makes subconscious decisions that influence their judgment and to help inoculate against their influence.

The remainder of the discussion included ways to minimize bias throughout the awards process. A key part of getting better representation of women among award winners is by increasing the pool of candidates. For example, some awards are given annually in fields with dwindling numbers of participants. Thus, it is important to rethink the timing of awards to generate larger pools from which to select the best nominees. When the nominations open, it is imperative to raise awareness by crafting solicitations that use gender-neutral language and then distributing them broadly through a variety of media, both print and online. Updating the organization's Web site to consolidate the location of the awards and their criteria on a single page, so that they are easy to find, is also encouraged. Creating canvassing committees and reaching out to women's and minority groups is another way to broaden the pool of nominees. Nomination and selection committees should also reflect the breadth and depth of the society's membership by ensuring gender and ethnic diversity. When these committees convene, they should begin by inoculating against implicit bias, discussing which specific qualities are to be evaluated, and disclosing any conflicts of interest so that the caliber of the nominees' credentials is what is being evaluated rather than the strength of their professional networks.

At the workshop's conclusion, each society developed its own list of best practices to suit the nature of its own discipline. These recommendations were taken back to the society for acceptance and ratification. The societies then implemented the changes accordingly and shared news of the project via their respective journals and member publications. AWIS tracked the progress of their awards program over the next 2 years and held a follow-up workshop in 2012 that included the 7 original pioneer societies as well as 11 new societies that approached AWIS after hearing about the project.

The outcome of the AWARDS project's first two years in regard to its intended goal of increased representation of women among award winners varied by society, as noted in Figure 8.22.

Sustainability from year to year remains a challenge and getting each society as a whole to fully and meaningfully embrace the importance of diversity, equity, and transparency—rather than just being able to check a box in a demographic survey—has sometimes been a stumbling block. However, AWIS's second objective, increasing the transparency of the awards process, has been met fairly successfully. A surprising number of other positive outcomes ensued as well. The American Mathematical Society increased the number of women in positions of leadership and on committees. The American Geophysical Union developed a computer program to identify networks of influence and connectivity to try to

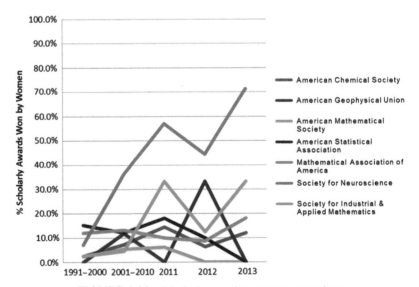

FIGURE 8.22   Scholarly awards to women over time.

minimize conflicts of interest, and the Society for Industrial and Applied Mathematics, in which women have been particularly poorly represented, increased the number of women on the editorial board for their 14 journals and doubled the number of women recognized as fellows. Finally, the Mathematical Association of America adopted a double-blind review process for their journals.

AWIS continues to track the trends of the 18 societies and is currently developing a Web site that will allow any society to enter its own statistics and thus evaluate the progress they are making toward gender equity in their awards process.

CONCLUSION

The following best practices are recommended to minimize the impact of bias in the interest of engineering a more inclusive and transparent scientific workplace:

- Inoculate against implicit bias by discussing it or showing an informational video before convening recruitment, tenure, and selection committees.
- When possible, mask the gender of candidates for positions.
- Encourage a double-blind review process for journal articles.
- Create heterogeneous committees that represent the breadth and diversity of the institution in terms of gender and ethnicity.
- Consider the influence of language when creating job solicitations and writing letters of recommendation as well as giving honorary names to awards, memorial lecture series, etc.
- When evaluating candidates for hiring, tenure, and other promotions, ensure that their accomplishments are being evaluated, not their qualities as individuals.

Government Policy Implications for Addressing Family-Related Issues

http://dx.doi.org/10.1016/B978-0-12-800215-5.00009-9

I would delay having children because I am unable to take maternity leave, and I fear that I would not find employment afterwards. —**A woman working in medicine and allied health, age 36–45 years, single, United Kingdom**

Sometimes I feel that most articles, even if they are interesting, will never change the way things are being done, or that changes are produced very slowly. —**A woman working in electrical engineering, age 26–35 years, married/partnered, Spain**

Family-friendly policies are essential to help retain women scientists, engineers, and technologists in the interest of strengthening diverse, competitive workforces and advancing a country's innovation enterprise, from academic institutions to disciplinary societies to nonprofit organizations to industrial sectors. Creating work environments where employees can balance the demands of career and family is good policy for both employers and employees; this assertion holds true across government, university, and industry work settings. The term "family-friendly policies" generally encompasses all workplace policies that foster a culture that accommodates the holistic, work/life dimensions of the workforce. Although often equated with the need for career flexibility arising from responsibilities associated with childbearing and child care, family-friendly policies should also encompass needs arising due to responsibilities associated with caring for elderly parents, sick partners, and adoptions.

THE UNITED STATES

The United States is one of four countries in the world that does not have a paid maternity leave policy. In stark contrast, many of the country's global competitors for the best and brightest minds lead the world in parental-assistance policies by offering 6 months or more in paid maternity leave.[87] There are many reasons besides inadequate maternity leave policies that lead women scientists, engineers, and technologists to choose to leave academia in particular. Attrition due to the difficulties of accommodating work and life has traditionally been higher for women, but with an increased trend toward more equitable distribution of child care and household responsibilities, more men are opting to leave for similar reasons. In the survey of more than 4000 male and female scientists from across the world reported in Chapter 2 of this book, one-third of all respondents admitted to struggling to balance their professional and personal lives.[88] Ten percent of respondents were considering a career change to better accommodate the demands of both home and work. Further, studies have shown that women with children are 28% less likely than women without children to get tenure and a staggering 35% less likely to get tenure than married men with children.[86]

The Family and Medical Leave Act

The need for family-friendly policies was initially perceived as a mechanism permitting trained female professionals to remain in the workforce. In recent years, this perception has expanded. It is now recognized that, in order for the United States to retain a competitive skilled workforce, the nation's employers must change their policies to make them more family friendly for both men and women. Such efforts have come from both employer-initiated changes in benefits and in response to legislation. A key piece of legislation that addresses at least a portion of the needs of employees with caregiving responsibilities, the Family and Medical Leave Act (FMLA), was signed into law in 1993. The law allows eligible employees (both women and men) to take up to 12 weeks of unpaid leave per year to support some family and medical needs. FMLA applies to employers with 50 or more employees; these employees are guaranteed continued health insurance benefits and employment in a position that is the same or equal to the one held prior to going on leave. While this law covers only about half of the total US workforce, it was an important first step in recognizing that approximately three-fourths of American children live in households where every adult in the home is employed. Unfortunately, even in organizations and institutions where family-friendly policies are endorsed and promoted, there often exist real or perceived biases against employees (regardless of gender) who use these benefits to balance their work/life responsibilities. This bias manifests in negative impacts on desirable work assignments/opportunities and promotions, with overall longer term impacts on career growth and employee retention. More important, employing organizations do not always promote and encourage use of the family-friendly policies guaranteed by FMLA to all employees, regardless of work sector or career level.

Overcoming bias directed toward individuals who avail themselves of family-friendly benefits will require cultural change and strong, visible leadership on this issue at the highest levels of organizations. Despite the profound importance of the groundbreaking FMLA legislation, research indicates that this law does not go far enough in ensuring that men and women who have significant caregiver responsibilities enjoy the support and flexibility required in order to reach their full potential in the workplace. One significant way in which FMLA benefits could be improved for workers involves expanding the definition of "family member" under FMLA to include, for example, siblings and domestic partners. Recent Supreme Court decisions will offer some relief in this regard with respect to domestic partners.

Paid Sick Leave

Another critical benefit needed by many employees with caregiving responsibilities is paid sick leave. In the United States, approximately one-half of all workers in the private sector have no paid sick leave benefit, resulting in significant financial burdens for workers who must take time off without pay to care for sick children and parents.[90,91] Research by Catalyst highlights the significant negative effect of parental stress associated with concern for the welfare of their school-aged children on workplace performance, career satisfaction, and cost to the employer. Specifically, Catalyst reports that approximately 2.6 million workers, male and female, are severely impacted by high anxiety about the welfare of their children (especially those in grades 6–12) after school, when they are often unsupervised. Employers who provided flexible work arrangements to accommodate parents' needs during this time of day saw positive effects on productivity, work performance, and employee satisfaction and retention. Finally, Catalyst reported that these stressors are gender neutral and have impacts on parents regardless of race and occupation level.[92]

Federal Grant-Funding Policies

A particularly troublesome obstacle to wide adoption of family-friendly practices in the United States has been the restrictive policies applied to recipients of federal funding for research and training support—policies under which money cannot be earmarked or used to help assist recipients in meeting family responsibilities while pursuing this work. The vast majority of science, technology, engineering, and mathematics (STEM) fields (and, increasingly, other sectors) in the United States are dependent upon such federal support for academically based work. Such structural impediments convey subtle yet strong messages to young men and women in their student years that the federal government and their institutions do not value other life responsibilities. Even those individuals or institutions that wish to provide such support have found their way blocked by federal grant policies or institutional rigidity in interpreting federal policy. Until very recently, US Federal Government policy has been both symbolically and pragmatically opposed to expenditure of federal dollars for anything deemed preferential to a particular class of recipients (say, parents) or for anything not directly related to the support of research (say, care support for children or elders).

In a small step forward in early 2013, the Office of Management and Budget (OMB) issued guidance on clarification of costs related to family-related leave and dependent care that may be charged to federal grants.[53] As noted by OMB,

> Existing guidance has long allowed recipient institutions to establish their own documented institutional policies around fringe benefits and travel, and to fund external meetings and conferences provided they meet the conditions established by the relevant item of cost. However, because family-related leave and dependent care are not discussed specifically in OMB guidance, there may be confusion over the documentation required to establish their allowability. In response, we have included specific language to clarify the requirements for documentation of these costs. This language does not require adoption of any new practices, and best mitigates risk of abuse of these policies by clearly aligning them with the existing requirement that any such costs are only allowable to the extent they are reasonable and consistent with written institution-wide policy and practice.

Under this new policy statement, family-related leave is an allowable fringe benefit under Section C-1; obtaining locally available dependent care resources for conference planning is an allowable cost under Section C-32, and temporary dependent care costs directly resulting from travel to conferences is an allowable cost under Section C-53.2.

This Federal Government effort to minimize one impediment to success is a step in the right direction. Moreover, these clarifications are an improvement on policy that will enable those who engage in this country's scientific enterprise to better accommodate the challenges of balancing life and work. Scientists, engineers, and technologists will be able to take family-related leave as well as to use grant funds to help cover the cost of care for children or elderly parents so that they can attend conferences. Attending conferences is crucial to facilitating the intellectual exchanges that are central to gaining academic tenure, promotion, and scientific jobs. Technical conferences provide a forum for networking with colleagues, creating new collaborative opportunities, disseminating one's research, and advancing one's career. Such exchanges also advance society at large in terms of the technology-transition process and the national interest in developing science capacity. However, the federal policies are contingent upon an institution-wide acceptance of the guidelines and are not implementable on a laboratory-by-laboratory basis. Therefore, a better policy would be to make this option available to anyone receiving these funds rather than tying them to university buy-in, which can be more difficult to achieve. Currently, only a handful of schools permit this use of federal funds, so few employees actually benefit. Furthermore, many small university laboratories are able to circumvent compliance with the FMLA because the law applies only to companies larger than 50 employees.

Minimizing the bureaucratic obstacles that distract from scientists' pursuit of research remains an important policy goal. Policies that enable scientists, engineers, and technologists to focus more of their attention on executing their work and less on navigating administrative hurdles are the most effective means by which the government can reap the benefits of its investment in the scientific enterprise. Therefore, a more permissive stance will be needed to make it easier for trained and talented people to continue to contribute to it.

Two federal agencies have initiated their own notable efforts to remedy some of the imbalances between the demands of a professional career and away-from-work life. The National Science Foundation launched a "Career-Life Balance" initiative that permits a no-cost extension of award duration for principal investigators on grants, which allows them to take an extended leave of absence to attend to dependent care responsibilities. Also, award funds may be used to temporarily replace project personnel who take leaves of absence because of such dependent care responsibilities, or to support additional personnel on the grant so as to sustain research when the principal investigator is on family leave.[93]

At the National Institutes of Health (NIH), meanwhile, grant funds may be expended for child care, parental leave, or additional technical support "provided such costs are incurred under formally established institutional policies that are consistently applied regardless of the source of support".[94] For trainees and fellows, up to eight work weeks of parental leave may be taken per year for the adoption or the birth of a child "when those in comparable training positions at the grantee organization have access to this level of paid leave for this purpose". Adjustments to appointment status may be requested in order to qualify for career-development awards to assist employees dealing with personal or family situations such as parental leave, child care, elder care, medical conditions, or a disability. For other family matters, applicants for funding can explain how personal circumstances may have delayed transition to an independent career or reduced scientific productivity; request an extension of eligibility to qualify as an early-stage investigator beyond 10 years, and/or apply for reentry supplements to ongoing grants. Applicants for conference grant support must include a description of the resources they need for child care and other types of family care at the conference site so that they may attend. Despite the many flexible options offered by the NIH, institutions still bear the responsibility for having family-friendly policies in place so that NIH grantees can take advantage of them.

Conclusions

To date, no common baseline of family-friendly benefits has been created across all federal funding agencies; the National Science Foundation and NIH policies represent a helpful, although limited, set of first efforts. In academia, hundreds of universities are proceeding with very little cooperation or agreement on accommodating family needs. The business sector has made somewhat more progress, recognizing the economic advantage of family-friendly benefits in attracting the workforce it needs.

EUROPE

The European Commission (EC) has been monitoring and maintaining a dataset on women in tertiary education and their advancement in science for the last 10 years, collecting data for all of their member states. The latest available data, for 2010, show that between 2002 and 2010, the remarkable growth in women's participation in higher education has now begun to produce visible impacts at the PhD level. In particular, the growth rates in the number of female PhD graduates in all countries in the European Union (EU) have been consistently higher than the number of men in all fields and subfields of science. In light of this progress, it is important to ensure that the investments in women's education and women's representation among doctoral candidates and recipients of PhD degrees do not decline. Fairness in recruitment and promotion is key, but equally important is the sensitivity of policy and decision makers to the needs and aspirations of both women and men in balancing their career and life responsibilities. The percentage of parents among the research population in Europe tends to be correlated with the percentage of parents in the working population at large, so that those countries with the highest/lowest proportion of researchers with children are also those with the highest/lowest proportion of parents in the working population. These findings underscore the centrality of work/life balance issues in the careers of female and male scientists.

In addition to gender equality policies that promote women's entry into the science labor market and address the quality of working conditions, policies specifically targeted at women in science are needed. A core need is to assure that motherhood does not preclude talented women from advancing in their academic career on the same terms as equally talented men. Science institutions must also translate these policies into practice. A key issue here is identifying better ways of recognizing and rewarding excellence that do not rely solely on the number of papers published and/or authorship status achieved during the early-career phase. A study by the European Molecular Biology Organization in 2010 has shown that even when the assessment and selection processes are "gender proofed", hidden gender bias in the criteria used, such as author status, results in more grants being awarded to men.[40] The consequence is that men gain more research grants, larger grants, and larger laboratories, while women have higher teaching loads—a disadvantage that establishes itself during the early-career stage and ripples through each next stage, growing in influence.

However, there has been a remarkable change in attitude toward gender issues in science as reflected in European policy during 2010–2012. Faced with the prospect of a shrinking working-age population and the challenges of creating sustainable growth after the financial crash of 2008–2012, scientists and policy makers have become more open to gender equality arguments as part of the solution.[39,40] One of the core goals of the EU, enshrined in the Treaty on the Functioning of the European Union, is to increase citizen participation in the labor force and, in particular, the employment of women.[95] Significantly, the EU's Europe 2020 strategy, devised to help Europe to emerge from the recent financial crisis, identified research and development as a major driver of sustainable economic growth and as a source of solutions to major societal challenges such as climate change, environmental preservation, and public health. To deliver on these expectations, all the available creativity and talent will be needed; the large pool of highly educated and skilled women represents ready-made human capital that must not be overlooked.

EU Policies and Human Capital

Increasing the number and excellence of researchers, as well as their mobility, are important aspects of the Europe 2020 strategy. A third aspect concerns researcher careers. In July 2011, the EC announced an investment in research and innovation (valued at approximately EUR 7000 million) as an economic stimulus to create 174,000 jobs as part of the European Research Area (ERA). The ERA is a policy tool for increasing the competitiveness of European research institutions via collaboration and encouraging more inclusive ways of working, including fostering greater mobility among knowledge workers.

However, if a united, Europe-wide research and development system is to emerge, many national and institutional barriers need to be dismantled first. Much of the policy effort has been directed at achieving the structural changes needed to improve the political governance of ERA, and at establishing partnerships with member states and among business, universities, and research organizations. The mobility of researchers is seen as critical to improving the flow of knowledge throughout

Europe by balancing demand for and supply of researchers in Europe, as well as leveling and improving these researchers' skills and career prospects.

The EC has promoted these goals through the Marie Curie Actions, a research fellowship program that includes a specific agenda for increasing the participation of women researchers by encouraging equal opportunities; designing actions to ensure that researchers can achieve an appropriate career/life balance; and making it easier to resume a research career after a break from work.[96] Other major initiatives include the European Charter for Researchers, a set of general principles and requirements that specifies the roles, responsibilities, and entitlements of researchers as well as their employers and/or funders, and EURAXESS—Researchers in Motion, an initiative providing access to a complete range of information and support services to researchers wishing to pursue their careers in Europe, or stay connected to it.[97]

These efforts extend the provisions for gender equality included in the Treaty on the Functioning of the European Union, which include "the Community shall aim to eliminate inequalities, and to promote equality, between men and women." The original scope of this objective was in formulating regulations on equal employment opportunity and equal work conditions in the EU; provisions included positive actions to achieve "equality in practice" (e.g., equal pay, equal access to employment including promotion, and equal access to vocational training, working conditions, and social security).

Interestingly, the original motivation for including gender equality among the core EU goals that resulted in the programs mentioned above was not the protection of fundamental rights to equal treatment, but rather to ensure competition on equal terms within the conditions that influence the performance of the internal (EU) market:

> The Community shall have as its task, by establishing a common market and an economic and monetary union and by implementing common policies or activities… to promote throughout the Community a harmonious, balanced and sustainable development of economic activities, a high level of employment and of social protection, equality between men and women, sustainable and non-inflationary growth, a high degree of competitiveness and convergence of economic performance, a high level of protection and improvement of the quality of the environment, the raising of the standard of living and quality of life, and economic and social cohesion and solidarity among Member States.

In other words, until 2010, the issue of gender equality in science was seen mainly as a factor in meeting the EU's economic goals, as a way to address the issue of underutilization of female talent. The Europe 2020 strategy focused on achieving smart, sustainable, and inclusive growth and extended the traditional view of gender equality by introducing research evidence that showed how gender inequalities in science can negatively impact women's careers and the quality and efficacy of research.

National Gender Equality Policies and Positive Measures

Since the 2006 introduction by Norway of quotas for women on company boards, the political discourse on gender equality in Europe has gained new energy, with the placement of women in top-level decision-making roles as the target of new policies. However, the Norwegian decision to target the gender composition of company boards was not made because boards were considered to be the most important arena for the exercise of power in the private economy; rather, it was driven by a perception that this was the only area in which regulation to change gender composition could be imposed.

Nevertheless, the Norwegian experience of implementing a legal quota requiring 40% of members of the corporate boards of public companies to be women has had a huge impact on the gender equality debate across many countries in Europe. Many different approaches have been implemented with a variety of objectives and scopes, influenced by each country's traditions and laws regarding corporations and shareholder rights; political makeup; and cultural attitudes toward gender equality.

The most common, and most modest, positive action promoted in Europe during this period has been a series of Gender Equality Action Plans. These plans are intended to promote policies, mechanisms, and values that should lead to greater opportunities for both women and men. Although weak in terms of impact because the approach fails to cover measures involving gender equality-related preferential treatment, Gender Equality Action Plans do go beyond the requirements imposed by antidiscrimination laws. A significant number of EU member states, such as the United Kingdom, Spain, Sweden, Austria, Italy, and the Netherlands, have opted to use this approach as a mandatory measure in public sector employment.

Gender Equality Action Plans have been widely adopted at universities and research organizations, and are seen as a useful, although lengthy, process by which to achieve structural change. However, their scope is not as ambitious as the United States' National Science Foundation-funded ADVANCE program. In particular, Equality Action Plans are conspicuous in their lack of reference to gender equality objectives that apply to the key functions performed by science institutions (training researchers and producing, applying, and communicating scientific knowledge). In 2013, it is therefore not surprising that, even in Norway, not one university has achieved the (voluntary) 30% target for women professors.

On a positive note, in 2012, two major EU-level policy initiatives, the aforementioned Horizon 2020 and ERA, have included gender equality in science practice and gender dimensions in research and innovation content as key criteria of success:

> The activities developed under Horizon 2020 should aim at promoting equality between men and women in research and innovation, by addressing in particular the underlying causes of gender imbalance, by exploiting the full potential of both female and male researchers, and by integrating the gender dimension into the content of projects in order to improve the quality of research and stimulate innovation. Activities should also aim at the implementation of the principles relating to the equality between women and men as laid down in Articles 2 and 3 of the Treaty on European Union and Article 8 TFEU.

> Gender equality and gender mainstreaming in research – to end the waste of talent, which we cannot afford, and to diversify views and approaches in research and foster excellence.

The EC has the tools to begin to promote implementation of these objectives, which include the provisions for action measures already encompassed by the EU legislative framework. The 40% target addresses the inclusion of the underrepresented sex in all expert groups, panels, and committees, and can be applied to the distribution of research funding under Horizon 2020.

Family Policies

In general, family policies in Europe are still marked by divergent approaches and differing preferences very much correlated with those nations' policies on "welfare" and employment. Left unresolved, these important issues can obstruct the EU goal of increasing researchers' mobility. A clear division exists between the Nordic and Anglo-Saxon countries, which have less explicit family policies focused more on individual rights and the welfare of the child, and the more conservative, Mediterranean, and postsocialist countries, which protect the family as a social unit, often through their constitutions. Significantly, as of 2009, only 10 of 27 EU countries had designated family ministries.

How Researchers Feel About Gender Roles and Their Careers

A survey of European doctoral candidates conducted in 2010 revealed many pressures experienced by young researchers, but in particular the feeling that they must postpone having children.[34] Surprisingly, this concern appeared to be the highest in the most "family-friendly" countries, such as Norway and Finland, which are typically portrayed as "female dominated". A majority of young researchers from these countries, including men, have reported strong pressure to postpone having children.

Conclusions

Important insights into the career/life tensions and pressures experienced by women and men are evident from surveys such as the doctoral candidate study described above. There appear to be a number of gender-role effects, linked to cultures and societal expectations and norms that influence how men and women feel about their careers. There is also much evidence of gaps between gender equality policies and their effective implementation into practice. For those in science careers, this lack of strategic implementation can create particularly difficult circumstances for reconciling career and life aspirations, as critical career development decisions and the need to demonstrate excellence tend to coincide with the timing of first parenthood. Policy makers and science institutions should pay attention to this issue if they are to succeed in their goals of recruiting and retaining a sufficient number of talented women and men. Effective support measures that are sensitive to family issues are particularly important in the early stages of science careers.

BRAZIL, CANADA, INDIA, AND SOUTH KOREA

The idea of a "family-friendly" workplace is a relatively recent phenomenon in many parts of the world, with varying degrees of progress demonstrated and where the modern is often combined with the traditional. The mix of policies and initiatives includes varying degrees of government-led, private sector-led, and traditional socioeconomic arrangements. A review of policies to support women in the workplace and in STEM fields in Brazil, India, South Korea, and Canada found similarities, although whether such policies are actually being implemented is not always clear or guaranteed. In this section, policies on maternity leave, child care, flexible work, and specific programs for women in STEM are compared. Also addressed is whether any of these nations' policies relate to research grants or breaks in employment. A substantial portion of the following analysis was undertaken in 2012 by Women in Global Science and Technology and the Organization for Women in Science for the Developing World with funding from the Elsevier New Scholars program.

Labor Force Participation

As in other countries discussed in this book, women's rates of employment and enrollment in science and technology fields are lower than men's employment in all four of the countries analyzed. Women's participation in the overall national labor force is a precondition for their participation in STEM areas, as well as influencing the domestic obligations that affect work/life balance for women in the workplace.

In South Korea, fewer than 50% of women are employed. This is one of the lowest rates in the developed world and is due primarily to social and cultural perceptions of women's role. Their participation in the labor force has been increasing over the past decade, although nonregular work makes up a large share of women's employment (approximately 40%) overall. This is also true for their employment in STEM, as discussed below. India sees an extremely low female to male labor force participation ratio at 35.9%, with less than 30% of women in the paid labor force in 2010. This proportion does not account for the percentage of women who work in the unpaid workforce as subsistence farmers, family workers, or microentrepreneurs. India has experienced a substantial drop in female labor force participation from 2000 to 2010, a result primarily of more women returning to school. However, this rate may also be affected by higher unemployment rates among women, causing them to drop out of the labor force entirely. Conversely, the female labor force participation rate in Brazil has been very high—at above 80%—for the past decade, although it dropped slightly between 2005 and 2010. In Canada, the participation rate of women in the labor force was 74.4% as of 2011, the highest rate of the past 21 years. The lowest rate of participation was 67.8% in 1993.

Women's Representation in Science and Technology

Due to lack of standardization of disaggregated data at all levels, the data selected to compare female participation in STEM sectors in the four countries were analyzed in three ways, grouping fields as follows: (A) natural and life sciences, engineering, and physics and natural sciences; (B) biology and medical and life sciences; and/or (C) engineering and physics including computer sciences.

The (A) category includes biology, medical science, nursing and pharmacy—in all of which women are highly represented—as well as all other scientific, technological, and engineering disciplines. The employment figures are highest (and rising) in India at 65.6%. Brazil shows less than half that rate, at 29.5%, as does Korea at 23.5%. Women's participation in these fields in India and Korea is rising, but Brazil experienced a drop from 32.4% to 29.5% over the decade (2000–2010).

As in the developed world, when category (A) is further divided into biology and medical and life sciences (category (B)) and engineering and physics (category (C)), the percentages are very different. If participation in engineering, physics, and computer sciences is dropped from the calculation, the ratio of women increases dramatically, to 44% in Korea, 70.1%

in Brazil, and a whopping 80.4% in India for the category (B) fields. The underrepresentation of women in physics, computer sciences, and engineering fields in these countries echoes the situation in the developed world. India shows the highest percentage of female enrollment in category (C) fields, at 35.8% in 2007. The percentage in Brazil was 20.8% for 2009, and in the Republic of Korea it was 14% for 2010. A positive sign is a trend of increasing percentages in each of these countries.

The data in Canada were divided into physical and life sciences and technologies; mathematics, computer, and information sciences; architecture, engineering, and related technologies; and agriculture, natural resources, and conservation. Percentages of women enrolling in postsecondary institutions in these fields of study were physical and life sciences and technologies, at 53.6%; mathematics, computer, and information sciences, at 24.2%; architecture, engineering, and related technologies at 17.5%; and agriculture, natural resources, and conservation, at 49.7%. These percentages show a slight drop from participation levels in 2005 and 2006.[98]

Rates of female participation in the STEM labor force dropped substantially in the four countries as females transitioned from completing their education to working, often by as much as 30 percentage points. In 2010, women made up 18% of the STEM labor force in Brazil, with India and South Korea at 12.5% and 12%, respectively, in 2008. As a comparison point, data from South Africa in 2004 showed a 16% participation rate by women in the STEM labor force. Interestingly, both Brazil and South Korea are unusual in that retention rates in the engineering and physics workforce are roughly commensurate with hiring rates. The reasons for this retention are not entirely clear; however, rates of enrollment in South Korea are also extremely low, so that systematic attrition may have occurred at earlier phases, such as during STEM education. For a variety of domestic and social reasons, the length of service of women in science and technology fields tends to be shorter than that of men, so that women's participation tends to decrease after entry into the workforce.[99] In the Republic of Korea, women's representation in the category of "science professionals and related jobs" has more than doubled, from 13.8% in 2001 to 31.4% in 2010. However, the revision of occupational classification during the same period could have influenced this increase as well. Further, female science professionals tend to be employed in less-than-full-time positions.[99] Some of the reasons for the positive retention rates in Brazil may include public and competition-based processes for filling positions in the university and national research system, a comparatively high representation of females in many science disciplines, and consistent public funding for tertiary and postgraduate students.[100]

From previous work, a South African study provides insight into the reasons for this drop in workforce participation, again similar to those seen in the developed world. A study of the participation of women in the industrial science, engineering, and technology sector for the South African Reference Group on Women in Science and Technology of the National Advisory Council on Innovation assessed responses to a questionnaire administered to 90 women in science, engineering, and technology companies across South Africa. Forty-six percent of these women worked in state-owned enterprises. The respondents identified the work environment as a key factor in facilitating or inhibiting women's participation in the STEM sector. Feedback on work performance, remuneration and promotion opportunities, gender relations in the workplace, race relations, mentorship and career development opportunities, and implications for family life of a career in STEM all played a role in determining women's participation in these industries. In-depth interviews with 38 senior women and company heads (CEOs) revealed additional factors affecting women's recruitment, retention, and advancement in industrial science and technology. These included the masculine image of science, gender-blind workplace policies with no emphasis on female constraints, the allocation of women into supportive roles, the challenge of balancing work and family responsibilities, gender discrimination and masculine organizational culture, sexual harassment, and the "glass ceiling".[101]

Data for Canada indicate that women comprise 44.6% of those employed in professional, scientific, and technical services, with women facing the same sets of challenges mentioned in South Africa.[102,103] While these numbers are quite high, as in other countries, women researchers in Canada are overrepresented in part-time positions and underrepresented at the highest levels, including in tenured positions.[103]

Domestic Responsibilities and Unpaid Work

While it is well recognized in most of the developed world that domestic responsibilities such as child care and housework are serious inhibitors of women's career advancement, in many countries of the developing world it is assumed that women are solely responsible for these and other unpaid duties. Subsistence farming, fetching water and firewood, and providing health care to their families are all unpaid activities and take up much of women's time. For this reason, the term "unpaid work" is used to refer to women's nonremunerative activities, to differentiate them from paid jobs and self-employment.

Women's doubled workday of family and professional responsibilities means they work, on average, longer hours than men worldwide.[104] They spend more time in unpaid work in all the countries discussed here, with the exception of Brazil—where available data indicate that men spend 30% more time in unpaid work than women. However, this disparity indicates some of the difficulty with comparable definitions, as Brazil has a separate category of "domestic work", in which women continue to spend substantially more time.[105] In a 2008 national pilot survey of time use, 86.3% of women interviewed said they did domestic work, while only 45.3% of men did so. Compared with 2001 data, it was found that the time spent on household work is declining for both men and women, with a greater decline for women. This trend is considered to be a result of new technology (access to water, electricity, and household equipment) and lifestyle changes (having fewer children, not returning home for lunch), which had a much stronger impact on women's workload. In 2001, women dedicated 29 h a week for domestic work; in 2008, the time commitment was 23.9 h. Men continued to dedicate fewer hours to these activities: in 2001, the time equated to 10.9 h a week and in 2008 to 9.7 h. The survey also showed that domestic work for men involved different tasks than for women. Men tend to work on outside chores such as gardening or washing the car, or on sporadic activities such as minor house maintenance.[100]

In India, women work longer hours than men and carry the major share of the household and community work that is unpaid. The system of national accounts shows an average workweek of about 42 h for men as compared with only 19 for women, but much of women's work does not show up in these statistics. Women spend nearly 10 times more time than men on household and care-related activities: about 2.1 h per day on preparing food and about 1.1 h on cleaning the household and utensils. Men's participation in these activities is nominal. Taking care of children is one of the major responsibilities of women, as they spend nearly 10 times the amount of time spent by men—about 3.16 h per week compared with 0.32 h. In learning, leisure, and personal care activities, males spend 8 h a week more than women.[106,107]

In South Korea, women spend more than five times the rate of men in unpaid work. In fact, the pattern in the South Korean labor market for women is gradual withdrawal due to childbirth and child rearing. Women withdraw from the labor market once they have children and generally do not return; recently they have begun to reenter the labor market once their children reach school age.[99]

Canadian women continue to spend more time than men on child care and domestic work, although the gap has been narrowing since the 1980s. In dual-income couples, the dominant family form in Canada since the 1980s, young adults are increasingly sharing economic and domestic responsibilities. As women have increased their hours of paid work, men have also steadily increased their share of household work. As well, hours of total housework have decreased. Nevertheless, from 2010 to 2011, women still spent approximately twice as many hours as men per week in caring for children and 13.8 h compared with men's 8.3 h per week on household domestic work.

Maternity Leave

All the countries examined here have a maternity leave policy of some sort. In Brazil, the Federal Constitution of 1988 expanded social rights, including provision of pregnancy and maternity leave, breaks for women workers to feed their babies, support for day care for up to six months, and paternity leave. Paid maternity leave is provided by the state only to a very small proportion of the population.

In Canada, both maternity/paternity leave and benefits are mandated for all employers, although benefits are paid through the national employment insurance plan. Depending on the length of employment and number of hours worked, new mothers can take between 17 and 52 weeks of leave from their jobs. Employers are required to keep their jobs available and they must resume providing the same rate of pay with the same employment benefits when the employees return. Maternity/paternity leave is paid for up to 15 weeks. Up to 55% of the average weekly wage (80% for low-income families) is paid out to a maximum amount. Employers are prohibited from discriminating against new hires for reasons of marital status or pregnancy.

The Indian Constitution includes provisions that the State is required to make provision for securing just and humane conditions of work and for maternity relief. Mothers are entitled to 12 weeks of paid leave, provided they have worked 80 days prior to the leave.

In South Korea, The Act on Gender Equality in Employment and Work-Family Reconciliation was amended in 2007 with the addition of clauses on maternity protection and work/family reconciliation, including parental leave for fathers, reduced working hours for mothers with young children, and division of maternity leave between mother and father. The provisions also include the requirement that employers provide education to prevent sexual harassment at work, establish and submit implementation plans for affirmative-action measures, grant child or family care leave, and reduce work hours to allow for child care. Paid leave is generous—parents are entitled to 90 days at 100% of their salary, followed by up to 1 year at 40% (up to a monthly maximum).

National Child Care Policy

The Republic of Korea appears to have the strongest policy on child care. Financial support has been maintained since the Infant Care Act in 2001. Of all households with children aged 0–5 years in 2009, the bottom 50% in income received full reimbursement for child care costs; households with incomes between the 50th to 60th percentiles were eligible for 60%, and households with incomes between the 60th and 70th percentiles were eligible for 30% of costs. At the end of 2008, 41.4% of children were provided child care services, and 64% of these children benefitted from child care grants.

India also has a policy, but it appears that child care facilities are not widely available. Some regions and states may institute programs. A recommendation made to the Indian Task Force on Women in Science was that day care/nursery facilities should be made available at research institutions. As a result of discussions with the Task Force, an announcement was made in 2008 that the Department of Science and Technology would provide financial support to institutions to provide child care facilities.[108]

In Brazil, some states or municipalities may provide local services. In principle, every firm of a certain size is obligated to offer child care facilities, but implementation of this policy is not widespread. For professional women in higher income groups, child care is included as part of hired domestic work. There are also many private nursery schools in urban areas. For lower income groups, the solution is found in the extended family—either a grandmother who provides day care or a young cousin or sister who is brought into the household to help out.

Canada lacks a comprehensive national child care program, although it was recommended by the Report of the Royal Commission on the Status of Women more than 40 years ago. The provinces of Ontario and Quebec offer early childhood education including all-day kindergarten, while Quebec also offers care for children up to 4 years old at a cost of just $7 per day.[109] Other provinces make available some degree of publicly funded day care—a certain number of spaces—to a lesser or greater extent. Child care costs can be deducted from personal income tax, and some provinces provide subsidies for private care.

Flexible Work Policy

None of the four countries have flexible work policies, although some countries have implemented incentives to promote flexi-work. In 2010, the government of South Korea implemented a work system that includes at-home work, telecommuting, and flextime for central and local government employees. One goal of the plan is to increase the number of women in the labor force to a rate closer to that of other Organisation for Economic Co-operation and Development countries. The plan includes five aspects of work: (1) the workplace, including at-home and telecommuting work, either at a smart office near the worker's residence or at a place outside the office using mobile devices; (2) hours, including flextime, selective work, compressed work, or discretionary work; (3) method, with core-time work; (4) dress, with a casual dress code; and (5) type, such as part-time work.[110] This plan has not gained momentum in the private sector, although a report in 2013 notes that less than 10% of Korean firms are implementing flextime practices.[111]

In India, the opposite pattern is taking place: flexible work practices have been gaining momentum in the private sector, yet no national government policy exists.[112,113] In 2008, the country's Department of Science and Technology announced it would support flexi-work in national science institutions.[108]

Brazilian labor law does not allow flexible work. All formal work contracts are full-time contracts. There is also currently no national law on flextime in Canada, although one province has implemented it at the provincial level. A recent federal court decision states that workplaces are obliged to accommodate reasonable child care-related requests from their employees. This judicial ruling may start a broader national discussion on work/family issues. Nevertheless, flextime and working from home are quite common practices in government, research, and the private sector.

Family-Friendly Policies and Programs for Women in Science

The countries examined here all recognize the importance of implementing family-friendly policies, although the degree of actual support varies considerably. With regard to family-friendly policies to support women in the scientific fields, there is much less concrete support in place. The South Korean Government has produced Basic Plans for Fostering and Supporting Women in Science and Technology every 5 years since 2004. These policies focus primarily on encouraging women and girls in the sector, including projects to encourage young women and girls to enter science and engineering, recruitment and promotion policies that target women, establishment of an "officer" in charge of women and gender issues at scientific institutions, providing research funds exclusively for women scientists in scientific institutions, and establishing an Institute on Women in Science and Technology. The one concrete, family-friendly initiative is the child care center (nursery school) established at Daedeok Research Complex in Daejeon. The complex employs 20% of the country's women scientists and engineers. The nursery school can accommodate 300 babies and toddlers between the ages of 15 and 60 months.[114]

The Indian Task Force on Women in Science has made a number of recommendations for family-friendly policies and programs to support women scientists, including (1) fostering and supporting the entrance of women into STEM employment through a supportive spouse policy and making available part-time jobs; (2) promoting career advancement and reentry through refresher training and mentorship for women who have had a break and wish to reenter the workforce; (3) removing age restrictions for women to participate in conferences/workshops, etc.; (4) supporting related issues at workplaces such as financial support for improvement of overall generic facilities such as toilets and safe transportation.[107] As has been noted earlier, the Indian Department of Science and Technology announced its intention to encourage research institutions to provide nursery facilities and support flexible work options for women scientists.[108]

Canadian data indicate that, compared with men, academic women tend to have fewer children, while those with children tend to be in lower academic positions than men with children. This is a result of the additional time women in academia spend on child care and other unpaid domestic labor. A survey of female Canada Research Chairs (the highest prestige research fellowship in Canada) showed that family or community responsibilities pose a large barrier for women researchers, rated second after barriers related to social capital and social schemas. Three main inhibitors emerged: family and child care responsibilities, parental leave, and mobility. To address these issues, many universities in the country provide day care facilities. Some implement "stop the tenure clock" policies, which enable tenure-track faculty to delay their tenure reviews because of family responsibilities or crises such as childbirth, adoption, or illness. Some universities implement spousal-hiring policies by offering relocation assistance to the spouses of new faculty. They may also offer tenured positions, contract-based positions, and nonacademic positions based on the merit of the potential spousal hire and the needs of the receiving university.[103]

Conclusions

Institutions in many of the countries examined here are taking some steps to support the family responsibilities of women, and in some cases to encourage men to take on some degree of domestic work and child care. This is happening through government policy, individual (and sometimes isolated) programs, and/or private sector practice. Solutions include paid and unpaid maternity and paternity leave (in some cases), and establishing child care programs either through national policy or institutional choice. Both the private sector and research institutions may institute the flexible workplace, allowing women to work from home, reduce their working hours, or bring their children to work with them. With uneven coverage through a patchwork of solutions continuing to be the norm in all countries, both developed and developing, one sees in developing countries an adherence to the traditional solutions of bringing in the extended family, choosing to drop out of the workforce to manage domestic tasks in accordance with societal trends, and hiring live-in domestic help.

SUMMARY

Developing and sustaining a viable community of STEM professionals is a challenge faced not only by individual countries, but also by all national and regional participants in the global marketplace. As noted in the analyses above, countries and global regions are beginning to recognize the necessity of moving toward gender equity and of developing policies that support full inclusion of both women and men in the STEM enterprise. In widely variant cultural contexts, the dilemma of early-to-mid-career scientists (especially women) is the need to balance family responsibilities with demanding academic careers (see Global Highlights below). Attrition rates among talented scientists caused by work/life issues must be addressed by implementation of policies that can provide sufficient flexibility for both workplaces and the individuals who are employed in them. To that end, the Elsevier New Scholars program has, through its funding, supported programs that encourage networking and collaborations among institutions and/or across STEM disciplines in ways that support the challenges of scientists with family responsibilities; develop and implement advocacy and policy development to retain, recruit, and develop women in science; and promote partnerships and knowledge sharing among institutions in the developed and developing world. There is still much work ahead. In academia, there has to date been very little cooperation or agreement on accommodating family needs. Business sectors have, however, begun to recognize the economic advantage of work/life and family-friendly benefits in attracting needed workforces. Introducing new ideas, capabilities, and capacity will remain a challenge for the foreseeable future. Model programs, such as those presented in this book, can provide guideposts on the way forward.

GLOBAL HIGHLIGHTS

China

- About 76% of Chinese researchers are satisfied with their career opportunities.
- About 41% of Chinese researchers state that they had delayed childbearing.

Japan

- Saying "no" to nonpriority projects was reported by 29% of Japanese researchers.
- One-quarter of Japanese researchers said that ensuring a good work/life balance has negatively impacted their careers.

United Kingdom

- Only 45% of UK researchers are satisfied with their work/life balance.
- Less than one-fifth of UK researchers (16%) indicated that there is sufficient support for their spouse/partner at their institution.

Germany

- Their balance between work and life is satisfactory for 51% of German researchers.
- About 58% of German researchers can delegate tasks to others in their workplaces.

The United States

- Only 13% of US researchers would consider moving to another country to further their careers.
- More than three-fourths (77%) of US researchers believe the work they are doing is making a difference to society.

France

- About 90% of French researchers undertake research because of the joy of discovery.
- Slightly more than one-quarter (27%) of French researchers have delayed having children to pursue their careers.

Canada

- About 61% of Canadians are comfortable saying no to work or projects that they do not consider a priority.
- Moving to another country to further career advancement is an interest of only 16% of Canadian researchers.

Italy

- About 60% of Italian researchers report satisfaction with their work/life balance.
- Only 46% of Italian researchers are satisfied with their career opportunities.

Spain

- About 61% of Spanish researchers are satisfied with their work/life balance.
- A desire to move to another country to further their career was reported by 32% of Spanish researchers.

Brazil

- About 78% of Brazilian researchers feel that their work is making a difference to society.
- Only 13% of Brazilian researchers report that ensuring a good work/life balance has negatively impacted their careers.

Appendix A. Roster of Participants and Meeting Agenda for "Rethinking the Future of the STEM Workplace: Convening of Global Experts on Work/Life Family Issues"

Michele Garfinkel, PhD, Manager, Science Policy Programme, European Molecular Biology Organization, Heidelberg, Germany

Joan Girgus, PhD, Professor of Psychology and Special Assistant to the Dean of the Faculty, Princeton University, Princeton, NJ, USA

Joan S. Herbers, PhD, Immediate Past President, Association for Women in Science, and, Professor of Evolution, Ecology, and Organismal Biology, Ohio State University, Columbus, OH, USA

Theodore Hodapp, PhD, Director of Education and Diversity, American Physical Society, College Park, MD, USA

Mary Anne Holmes, PhD, Professor of Practice, and Director, ADVANCE Nebraska, University of Nebraska, Lincoln, NE, USA

George Kamkamidze, MD, PhD, Head of the Board, Maternal and Child Care Union, Tbilisi, Republic of Georgia

Christine Littleton, JD, Vice Provost for Diversity and Faculty Development, and Professor of Law and Women's Studies, University of California—Los Angeles, Los Angeles, CA, USA

Kelly Mack, PhD, Program Director, ADVANCE Program, National Science Foundation, Arlington, VA, USA

Sandra Masur, PhD, Past Chair, Women in Cell Biology, Professor of Ophthalmology, and Associate Professor of Structural and Chemical Biology, Mount Sinai School of Medicine, New York, NY, USA

Angela Doyle McNerney, BA, President and Executive Director, TechValleyConnect, Rensselaer Technology Park, Troy, NY, USA

Elizabeth Pollitzer, PhD, Chief Executive Officer, Portia Ltd, London, United Kingdom

Maria Santore, PhD, Director and Professor of Polymer Science and Engineering, University of Massachusetts-Amherst, Amherst, MA, USA

Barbara Silver, PhD, Assistant Research Professor of Psychology and ADVANCE Program Director, University of Rhode Island, Kingston, RI, USA

Cindy Simpson, CAE, MEd, Director of Programs and External Relations, Association for Women in Science, Alexandria, VA, USA

Gerlind Wallon, PhD, Deputy Director, European Molecular Biology Organization, Heidelberg, Germany

ELSEVIER AND ASSOCIATION FOR WOMEN IN SCIENCE PARTICIPANTS

Janet Bandows Koster, CAE, MBA, Executive Director and Chief Executive Officer, Association for Women in Science, Alexandria, VA, USA

Keisha Byrd, Director of Meetings and Special Events, Association for Women in Science, Alexandria, VA, USA

Donna J. Dean, PhD, Executive Consultant and Past President, Association for Women in Science, Alexandria, VA, USA

Susan Fitzpatrick, PhD, President, Association for Women in Science and Vice President, James S. McDonnell Foundation, St. Louis, MO, USA

David Ruth, MA, Senior Vice President, Global Communications and Executive Director, Elsevier Foundation, New York, NY, USA

Ylann Schemm, MA, Program Manager, Elsevier New Scholars Program, Elsevier Foundation, New York, NY, USA

AGENDA

WEDNESDAY, MARCH 7, 2012

8:30 a.m.	Welcome and Opening Plenary • Susan Fitzpatrick, President, Association for Women in Science • David Ruth, Executive Director, Elsevier Foundation • Donna J. Dean, Consultant, Association for Women in Science
10:00 a.m.	Coffee and networking break
10:30 a.m.	Panel 1—Dual Careers and Strategic Decision Making • Thought leader and panel moderator—Joan S. Herbers, Ohio State University • Tech Valley Connect—Angela Doyle McNerney, President and Executive Director • Portia Ltd—Elizabeth Pollitzer, CEO
11:45 a.m.	Panel 2—Addressing Work/Life Issues • Thought leader and panel moderator—Mary Anne Holmes, University of Nebraska • Association for Women in Science—Cindy Simpson, Director of Programs and External Relations • Maternal and Child Care Union—George Kamkamidze, Head of the Board
1:00 p.m.	Working lunch and networking
2:15 p.m.	Panel 3—Child care/Dependent Care in Professional Contexts • Thought leader and panel moderator—Michelle Garfinkel, European Molecular Biology Organization • European Molecular Biology Organization—Gerlind Wallon, Deputy Director • American Physical Society—Theodore Hodapp, Director of Education and Diversity • American Society for Cell Biology—Sandra Masur, Mount Sinai School of Medicine
3:30 p.m.	Panel 4—Promoting Family Friendly Policies • Thought leader and panel moderator—Kelly Mack, National Science Foundation • University of Massachusetts Amherst—Maria Santore, Director • University of California, Los Angeles—Christine Littleton, Vice Provost for Diversity and Faculty Development • Princeton University—Joan S. Girgus, Professor of Psychology • University of Rhode Island—Barbara Silver, ADVANCE Program Director
4:45 p.m.	Closing remarks for day • Donna J. Dean, Executive Consultant and Past President and Janet Bandows Koster, Executive Director and CEO, AWIS
6:00 p.m.	Reception at United Nations

THURSDAY, MARCH 8, 2012

8:00 a.m.	Working breakfast—Review of previous day by Donna J. Dean
	• Perspectives from previous day's panels
9:00 a.m.	Roundtable Discussions (breakout groups led by thought leader/panel moderator)
	• Cross-cutting groups of attendees addressing effective strategies for broader and more comprehensive implementation and sustainability of programs
10:30 a.m.	Group share and summary
	• Moderated by Donna J. Dean and Ylann Schemm, Program Director, Elsevier New Scholars Program
11:30 a.m.	Next steps
12 p.m.	Adjourn meeting
12:15 p.m.	Lunch
	Press briefing
	Individual interviews with participants
3:00 p.m.	Conclude press event

Appendix B. Overview of Elsevier Foundation New Scholar Project Awards by Year

Awardee: Princeton University

Project title: Dependent Care Program for Graduate Students and Post-doctoral Fellows in Science and Engineering.

Original goal: To establish a fund that provides travel grants to graduate students and postdoctoral fellows in the natural sciences and engineering who are parents of young children, to allow them to attend academic conferences and other career-building events.

Award period: One year.

Accomplishments: The Elsevier award was used as seed funding for a new program modeled upon the institution's dependent-care travel fund for faculty. Awards were used by graduate students and postdoctoral recipients for dependent care at a conference or at an alternative location and expenses could include those incurred in transporting a caregiver.

Sustainability: In September 2007, Princeton University submitted a follow-up proposal to the refocused New Scholars program to extend and expand the coverage of the above award to postdoctoral fellows. (See 2007 Awards section below for information on that project.)

Awardee: Society of Toxicology

Project title: Distinguished Woman in Toxicology Award.

Original goal: To establish and fund an annual award over 3 years to recognize a "Distinguished Woman in Toxicology". An annual award of $3300 will be presented to an individual (male or female) in academia, government, industry, or a related field who has been a major influence in the mentoring of women scientists entering the field of toxicology and/or whose leadership and service have provided career-development opportunities for women toxicologists or encouraged women to achieve their professional goals.

Award period: One year, but used to support three years of activities.

Accomplishments: The first annual award was made to Linda Birnbaum in March 2008, followed by Yvonne Wan in 2009 and Curtis Klaassen in 2010.

Sustainability: The Elsevier Mentoring Award was awarded for three years, and the Women in Toxicology Special Interest Group of the Society of Toxicology is continuing the "Women in Toxicology Mentoring Award" on an annual basis.

Awardee: Boston University

Project title: Women in Science and Engineering Initiative.

Original goal: To support a graduate engineering student from Lebanon (Tala Succari) in the Department of Electrical Engineering and workshops of the WISE initiative. However, Ms Succari, following a change of advisor and later institution, was unable to accept the New Scholars program grant awarded to her. The Women in Science and Engineering (WISE) committee planned to select an appropriate replacement candidate, but none were identified. In August 2010, WISE requested permission to use the award for a series of WISE research networking workshops.

Modified goal: To support women faculty through a series of research and networking workshops that are intended to foster new research collaborations and the formation of small interacting groups.

Award period: One year.

Accomplishments: Not applicable at this time.

Sustainability: Not applicable at this time.

Awardee: University of California, Berkeley

Project title: The Open Sesame Project: IT Access for all Literacy Levels in Developing Regions.

Original goal: To support Dr Madelaine C. Plauché (PhD, linguistics, UC Berkeley), a postdoctoral field researcher at the International Computer Science Institute, in deploying the Open Sesame Project Toolkit in four village centers in Tamil Nadu, India, as part of the "Big Ideas @ Berkeley" program, which supports young scholars in implementing community programs.

Award period: One year.

Accomplishments: The Open Sesame application user interface system allows local experts to address specific needs in any domain by disseminating relevant, local-language digital materials in a form that is accessible to all individuals, even those with limited literacy skills.

Sustainability: The open-source nature of the technology should lead to further innovation and adaptation to new organizations, new languages, and new domains.

Awardee: University of California, Berkeley

Project title: Science, Technology and Engineering Policy Group (STEP).

Original goal: To support Dr Kathryn Hammond (doctoral student in bio-engineering) in development of training programs that provide scientists with skills to communicate effectively and understand decision-making processes of political institutions, as part of the "Big Ideas @ Berkeley" program, which supports young scholars in implementing community programs.

Award period: One year.

Accomplishments: STEP hosted an on-campus speaker series, ran a science and technology—policy white paper competition, and awarded travel grants to members to meet with federal science policy makers. More than 40 students participated in the white paper competition, with four finalists presenting their proposals to a public audience.

Sustainability: The white paper competition and speaker series will continue with benefactor funding. The first science and technology policy symposium in August 2008 featured presentations from the travel-grant program recipients funded by the Elsevier award.

Awardee: California Institute of Technology

Project title: Functional roles of WNT and SNAIL2 Target Genes in the Neural Crest.

Original goal: To support senior postdoctoral work of Dr Lisa Taneyhill (PhD, molecular biology, Princeton) in the laboratory of Dr Marianne Bronner-Fraser for a fifth year.

Award period: One year.

Accomplishments: The work resulted in a paper entitled "Functional roles of WNT and SNAIL2 target genes in the neural crest" published in *Developmental Biology* in December 2007. The additional research time also aided Dr Taneyhill in securing a tenure-track faculty position at the University of Maryland in 2007.

Sustainability: In her faculty position, Dr Taneyhill will continue her research on the functional significance of specific target genes during neural-crest emigration.

Awardee: Keio University

Project title: Day Nursery Program.

Original goal: To establish a daycare program at Keio University to support women scholars in their efforts to balance child care responsibilities with the demands of an academic career at one of Japan's most prestigious universities.

Award period: One year.

Accomplishments: The recognition from the Elsevier Foundation was sought to help commemorate Keio University's 125th anniversary.

Sustainability: Unknown.

2007 AWARDS

Awardee: Rensselaer Polytechnic Institute

Project title: Tech Valley Connect (Formerly PhD Move and SettleNet).

Original goal: To address barriers to relocation affecting the recruitment and retention of new women scholars, particularly those with working spouses and partners, by establishing resources such as relocation counseling, a regional career network for faculty spouses, and career coaching for both the scholar and the spouse.

Award period: Three years.

Accomplishments: During the three-year term of the grant, Tech Valley Connect developed an innovative start-up regional consortium of academic institutions and businesses aimed at improving recruitment and retention of both prospective and new PhD-holding and professional employees by focusing on dual-career challenges. Tech Valley Connect addresses barriers to relocation that affect the recruitment and retention of new women scholars, particularly significant in that research suggests that the number one reason universities and industry are unable to hire or retain high-level employees is the failure of their partners and families to successfully relocate. The program was presented at the annual Dual Career Conference at the University of Iowa, Iowa City in June 2010 to share best practices about Tech Valley Connect's consortium model. The group has also regularly received queries from other universities.

Sustainability: The initial pilot program (PhD Move) was officially concluded on December 31, 2009 with the formation of Tech Valley Connect's new Board of Directors (12 senior leaders from the organizations that participated in the pilot program, the President of the Albany/Colonie Chamber and representatives from the Center for Economic Growth) and the transition to nonprofit status achieved on January 4, 2010. Key elements of the new organization are the intent to: build a cost structure that will support the organization, identify new sponsorship opportunities, expand membership, continue outreach activities and ongoing support of informational networking interviews, build a members-only Web site, and hire a team of highly networked relocation specialists or "concierges" capable of customizing a relocation package for individual families.

Awardee: Princeton University

Project title: From Graduate Student to Assistant Professor: Helping Postdoctoral Scientists and Engineers Meet the Demands of Career and Family Life.

Original goal: To focus on the postdoctoral period in addressing two key needs: funding for a dependent-care travel program for postdoctoral fellows and travel support for fellows whose spouses are graduate students or postdoctoral fellows in science and engineering at another institution.

Award period: Two years.

Accomplishment: As the institution gained experience with the two grant programs, they discovered that they had considerably underestimated the need for its Spouse/Partner Travel Program grants and overestimated the need for its Dependent Care Travel Fund grants, and therefore funds were redistributed to the program of higher demand. In addition, the Princeton administration further supplemented the funding for the Spouse/Partner Travel grants to the humanities and social sciences postdoctoral communities. A total of 27 awards were made, and recipient surveys conducted. Two key findings emerged: (1) the grants reduced the amount of recipients' stress, permitting a greater ability to focus on their research programs and (2) the structure and organization of the program worked effectively.

Sustainability: Princeton developed a comprehensive and effective approach for publicizing, implementing, assessing, and modifying these new travel programs. There is a clear intent to continue the programs, but no specific plans or committed funds have been identified.

Awardee: Computability in Europe Conference Series, Coordinated by University of Amsterdam

Project title: Increasing Representation of Female Researchers in the Computability Community.

Original goal: To increase the representation of women researchers in all categories at CiE events (program committees, keynote speakers, session organizers, session speakers, contributing speakers) by implementing four main program elements (child care, workshops, a mentoring system, and incentives) at CiE conferences in 2008 (Athens), 2009 (Heidelberg), and 2010 (Ponta Delgada).

Award period: One year; used to support three years of activities.

Accomplishments: Following North American conference models, CiE implemented a new mentoring system in 2008 that enabled 16 women graduate students to develop strong ties with three senior women scientist/mentors. In addition, the 2008 Women in Computability workshop raised awareness of the problems that young female researchers are encountering and provided examples of successful research careers. In order to increase the percentage of women speakers (keynote, special session organizers, and contributing speakers) at CiE to 25% by 2010, the project team is eliciting increasing numbers of applications from women, but noted that much more work will be needed. The incentives program (providing financial support to conference organizers to invite senior female speakers) was not implemented due to the reduced project budget.

Sustainability: The mentoring system and the workshop were continued for the 2009 and 2010 meetings, but the free child care will be dropped if no participants are interested. Whether incentives for senior, midcareer, and junior female researchers could be implemented was still under consideration. For CiE in 2011, modest travel support was to be available and the Women in Computability workshops were anticipated to continue.

Awardee: American Society for Cell Biology

Project title: A Sustainable System for Supporting Child Care at the ASCB Annual Meeting.

Original goal: To establish a three-year program of competitive financial awards that will cover child care costs, permitting qualified ASCB members to attend the annual meeting, with a plan to sustain the awards beyond the period of support by establishing working relationships with the home institutions of ASCB members.

Award period: One year, for support at three successive annual meetings.

Accomplishments: The ASCB succeeded in creating a three-year child care and travel-grant program from this award (substantially scaled down from their initial funding request). Activities included: the selection of an awards committee; the design of an advertisement; application form and grant assessment survey; the review and selection of applications by the awards committee; media outreach; the annual meeting; and follow-up assessment with grant winners. The results of the program have proven overwhelmingly positive in the postmeeting surveys. Half of all respondents reported that they would have been unable to attend or would have experienced the conference as a financial burden without this critical support. All grantees were required to present abstracts at the meeting, which offered extensive networking opportunities with other scientists. Ninety-five percent of them reported that the meeting had been extremely helpful to their careers. This program demonstrated strong organization and media outreach, institutional commitment, and maximum award impact within a limited budget.

Sustainability: The ASCB sought sustainable funding options after 2010 and the program has continued at the annual meetings.

Awardee: University of Rhode Island

Project title: Transitional Support Program.

Original goal: To create and disseminate a series of programs to help new scholars in science, technology, engineering, and mathematics meet both their academic and parental obligations while on the job. The centerpiece of the initiative was the development of a model lactation program, which intended to establish a prototype lactation room and advisory resources for lactating faculty mothers.

Award period: Three years.

Accomplishments: The Elsevier Transitional Support Program at the University of Rhode Island enabled the university to launch and disseminate a model lactation program for student, staff, and faculty new mothers returning to work. Related goals included developing a work/life regional consortium providing support services to new mothers (particularly junior women in science, technology, engineering, and mathematics (STEM)) and winning the Rhode Island "Breastfeeding Friendly Workplace" gold award. Five lactation rooms were opened. Literature was disseminated and the program coordinator conducted a campus needs assessment and researched, wrote, and disseminated a University lactation policy in January 2009 to ensure that workers would be able to use the facilities without negative consequences. As well, meetings were held with the Rhode Island Department of Health Breastfeeding Coalition to disseminate information and with key personnel at institutions of higher education across the state. These meetings also served to launch a regional consortium and contact with nearby schools outside Rhode Island.

Sustainability: The goal of developing supplementary support services has been largely realized through a well-supplied lending library, strong ties to three community lactation consultants, and a series of informational lunches. A regional work/life consortium listserv is being established for promotion of collaborative events and meetings, as is a Work/Life Web site. The principal investigators continue to give presentations and anticipate submitting a paper for publication.

Awardee: University of California, Irvine

Project title: Professional Development Grants for Parents of Infants and Toddlers.

Original goal: To develop a targeted program to help scholars with family responsibilities attend professional conferences and events, and encourage them to continue their contribution to scientific discovery and innovation.

Award period: Three years.

Accomplishments: The program provided dependent-care assistance to faculty who are at least 50% responsible for child care in their families in order to demonstrate that career excellence and healthy families are not mutually exclusive aspirations. Over the three-year grant period, the total number of grants was 78, each capped at $1000. The awards were used for child and/or caregiver travel as well as to provide augmented child care services due to an absent caregiver. Faculty recipients attended or presented research at both domestic and international conferences in 2009. While the majority of recipients were assistant professors, associate professors also benefited from the program.

Sustainability: The program's steady growth in applications and usage reports has proven that the program is highly valued. An external evaluation of the award program is being assessed as to whether the program (1) raised awareness about the commitment to work/life balance and (2) diminished any perceived or real stigma associated with the use of these family friendly resources. The institution will share their experience with other institutions in California.

Awardee: University of Illinois at Urbana-Champaign

Project title: Encouraging Diversity and Work/Life Balance in Engineering Faculty.

Original goal: To create a monthly forum for faculty and postdoctoral students and their families to provide social reinforcement, advice, and peer counseling as a means to increase the advancement of women faculty in technical fields through recruitment and retention programs, spousal-hire programs, and awareness building.

Award period: One year.

Accomplishments: The project began in fall 2008, dedicated to assisting young engineering faculty (i.e., tenure-track faculty with less than five years' service) in managing work/life issues and forming a connection to the university and the local community. Postdoctoral fellows were also included, bringing the target group to approximately 100 (the College of Engineering has a faculty totaling approximately 400). Rather than arranging seminars on time management or creating brochures about community resources, the university gave faculty the chance to meet one another and engage with the community. Response has been very positive, although it has been challenging to reach and involve a large number of the new faculty. Interest is high, but time commitments and work pressures make it difficult for these busy professionals to "take a break". Young faculty and postdoctoral researchers welcome these events and view them very positively, even if they may not be able to participate in all of them. The beginnings of some social and professional connections have been formed between attendees, and it is hoped that these can be continued and widened.

Sustainability: No information was provided on how the program would be continued after the funding period.

2008 AWARDS

Awardee: Maternal and Child Care Union, Tbilisi, Georgia

Project title: A Program for Personal and Professional Development of Women Scientists in Georgia.

Original goal: To create a framework of national issues, capacities, mentoring, and support for women scientists in Georgia.

Award period: One year.

Accomplishments (from final report): At the beginning of the project, a survey of 100 Georgian postdoctoral women candidates identified key issues, which led to the development of a week-long training course that covered a broad range of topics. One hundred and fifty-three Georgian women scientists from different regions and institutions learned to use the tools, skills, and networks needed to advance their careers including developing grant proposals, managing research projects, publishing results, successfully balancing work and family, and assuming leadership positions. The final results of the survey and training project were presented to representatives of Georgian academic and research institutions, the media, and policy makers, and members of parliament. In addition, a national TV broadcast interview about the program was conducted by the Georgian Ministry's Deputy Chief of the Health and an article highlighting the survey results and the project's achievements was published in *Modern Medicine*, Georgia's most popular medical journal.

Sustainability: The publication above included conclusions and recommendations and a Web site was developed to archive the lecture materials for access by interested individuals and institutions for educational purposes.

Awardee: Association for Women in Science

Project title: Leading Women to Create Their Own Definition of Work/ Life Satisfaction.

Original goal: To develop and facilitate an educational/support program on work/life balance, including a toolkit with supplementary resources and extended coaching. The objective of the work/life program was to give women in STEM the tools they needed to achieve their personal work/life balance.

Award period: Three years.

Accomplishments: The Association for Women in Science (AWIS) workshop was pilot tested in nine AWIS chapters across the country, reaching

342 women scientists. In parallel, AWIS conducted a survey of 409 members, revealing that 68% of respondents reported that work/life balance issues had a definite impact on their decision to have or delay having children. Seventy percent reported not taking advantage of or having access to work/life balance resources at all. Hence, the workshop was refined to focus on helping women researchers examine how their current choices affect their work/life satisfaction and identifying the changes that will have the biggest impact on their professional and personal development, productivity, and performance.

Based on ongoing participant feedback and focus group feedback, content was refined and program length modified. The program was re-titled "Work/Life Satisfaction", as the notion of "balance" was highly disputed by workshop attendees. Concurrently, program materials for a "Program in a Box" toolkit for chapters were developed, including: a facilitator's instruction guide, a workshop outline, a PowerPoint presentation, a participant workbook, promotional material, participant self-evaluation instruments, and program evaluations. As an additional benefit to AWIS members who participated in the on-site educational program, fee-based group coaching sessions were offered to participants who would like to deepen their learning experience. There was a low response rate to the availability of follow-up coaching. More women were interested in follow-up peer mentoring, either in-person or virtual, and additional consideration was given to developing a peer-mentoring network as a way for individuals to stay connected and to continue to network with each other.

In the second year of the project, the program was presented to 14 additional AWIS chapters and at three different scientific society meetings reaching approximately 600 additional individuals across the country. As AWIS entered the third year of the project, continued outreach was accomplished utilizing the AWIS chapters across the United States in combination with targeted outreach to various professional scientific societies. Evaluations were conducted each time the program was presented, and modifications were made along the way to make the program more relevant for individuals in STEM. The changes that were made (e.g., adding case studies, making it more gender neutral, and referencing other research studies) were well received by the participants, which include the need for a more gender neutral presentation, as well as for broadening the presentation to individuals outside of the scientific community, resulted from observations made by the workshop presenters. A number of inquiries were made as to the focus of the program (was it just for scientists?) as well as the gender of the participants (was it just for women?). Over time, an increase in the number of individuals representing the other STEM fields (engineering, technology, and mathematics) and men in attendance required further modifications to the program, which resulted in a more robust presentation.

The combined number of individuals who benefited from attending the work/life satisfaction program over the past three years was more than 2500. The success of this program is attributable to the fact that it was data driven and was specifically developed by scientists for scientists. Although the original focus was on women scientists, the program now includes men as well. The program has also been expanded beyond scientists to include engineers, technologists, and mathematicians, as many of these individuals are also facing challenges relating to work/life satisfaction.

Sustainability: To sustain the program after the project period, 30 chapter leaders were convened for a two-day Work/Life Satisfaction session and received professional development, train-the-trainer instruction, and program branding guidance. To date, 16 AWIS chapters have presented the Work/Life Satisfaction program at least once, and more sessions are planned. The workbook and resource guide providing suggested readings and Web sites focusing on the topic of work/life satisfaction are also available on the AWIS Web site for access by AWIS chapter leaders. The formal presentation is available in a number of versions to best meet the specific needs as well as the time constraints that may exist in presenting this program on a local level. An e-workbook containing exercises for self-reflection and ongoing assessment based on what was learned during the on-site programs can be distributed to all participants to help them to identify areas they need to address within their work and home lives. Webinars and online networking resources were implemented to support ongoing learning for participants of local programs and beyond. Online discussion forums are active and training webinars are available on the basic components of the program to continue the discussions after the initial training has been completed.

AWIS has continued its outreach and participation in other scientific events and meetings to promote the findings and effectiveness of the workshop approach. The program has been very well received by the participants in a number of settings, and modifications can be made based on continuous assessment and evaluation. The program is very adaptable to meet the needs of the audience. A significant strength is that it is very interactive, which encourages participants to share their stories and to learn from each other both during and after the program. Based on the lessons learned, AWIS is considering the potential for implementation of the work/life content planning survey on an international scale. The survey instrument is robust and could be used to further investigate issues facing women in the corporate arena, in the academy, and by career level. Many survey questions could be adapted and used to further investigate issues facing individuals in the STEM field. Although originally there was a low response rate to the coaching program, AWIS is reevaluating its approach; coaching has become an important aspect for professional success for many scientists and provides them with the ability to make important decisions in a more objective manner.

The development of a worldwide mentoring platform is also under consideration. Research has shown that mentoring provides a much higher level of satisfaction and job retention for individuals in STEM and is important not only in the United States, but also for individuals, particularly women, around the world. Many women scientists are struggling with overcoming antiquated ideas on the role of women in universities, corporations, and government agencies. Successful mentoring by senior-level women who could provide career advice based on their own experiences would help to benefit these struggling scientists. In exchange, these senior-level women would be able to give back to their profession by sharing their knowledge and expertise. A critical facet here is an examination of the feasibility before proceeding further.

Awardee: Society for the Study of Evolution, Society of Systematic Biologists, and American Society of Naturalists, Coordinated by University of the Pacific and Museum of New Zealand Te PapaTongarewa

Project title: Child Care and Mentoring Support at the Annual Evolution Conference.

Original goal: To provide an integrated approach to child care and mentoring needs at the annual evolution conference (on-site, subsidized child care services; a professional mentoring program for 50 to 100 pairs administered through MentorNet; and a themed keynote lunch symposium).

Award period: One year, to support activities at three sequential annual meetings.

Accomplishments: The Evolution 2009 Conference successfully delivered not only a child care and mentoring program, but also a survey to analyze the results. Year one of the grant absorbed 44% of the funds, in line with the plan to steadily decrease subsidies over the three-year period to ensure sustainability and coverage by the three societies at the end of the grant period. Year two (Evolution 2010) featured child care, increased outreach regarding the MentorNet activities, and the luncheon symposium program presented by the Association for Women in Science, another New Scholars grantee, on their own Elsevier-supported project.

Sustainability: The three sponsoring societies committed support for continuing costs of on-site, professional child care, the professional mentoring program administered through MentorNet, and an annual luncheon symposium on issues of importance to retaining women and minority scientists in academia as well as research for the annual evolution conferences in subsequent years.

Awardee: Committee on the Status of Women in Physics, American Physical Society

Project title: Support for Child Care at American Physical Society (APS) Annual Meetings.

Original goal: To provide funds to young physicist parents for child care support consistent with making APS meetings a more family friendly environment and to develop a program intended to be a model for the adoption of similar programs for other physics conferences and institutions.

Award period: Three years.

Accomplishments: Attendance at the APS meetings is a key part of networking within the community and a source of professional support for physicists in smaller, more isolated environments. On-site and at-home child care-support stipends were offered for each of the two major conferences in 2009 (Pittsburgh and Denver) and 2010 (Washington, DC and Portland, Oregon.) A parent–child quiet room was provided at the Pittsburgh site in addition to onsite child care arrangements and local daycare providers. Priority was given to physicists in early stages of their careers. The funds augmented those already pledged to this purpose by the APS. Requests for grants increased significantly in 2010 due to additional advertising.

Sustainability: The APS allocated $5000 in 2008, 2009, and 2010 for child care grants as a pilot program. This was an experimental program and had not been a continuing commitment. Based on the data on usage of the proposed program collected through the enhanced Elsevier-supported program, the APS expects to continue to offer these grants in coming years in order to address the financial disadvantage that parents responsible for child care (mostly women) may face in attending meetings, which are essential in a successful career. As this program is advertised and utilized in coming years, usage of these resources is expected to increase. The program's aim is to influence the culture of the field, which is shifting from a model of traditional male breadwinners to one where both parents share family responsibilities.

Awardee: European Molecular Biology Organization

Project title: Child Care at the European Molecular Biology Organization (EMBO) Meeting.

Original goal: To fund child care facilities at the annual EMBO life sciences conference.

Award period: One year.

Accomplishments: Subsidized multilingual, on-site child care services were offered at the 2009 EMBO conference venue in Amsterdam, attended by more than 1300 participants from 50 countries. This program directly enabled young European life scientists to take full professional advantage of the EMBO conference and served as a family friendly model among scientific societies in Europe. During the conference, EMBO worked with a licensed child care provider and nature educator that embedded life sciences themes into the children's daily activities through explorations of the city's parks and museums. The anticipated 35-Euro per day per child fee was absorbed by the grant because of the lower-than-anticipated turnout numbers comprising nine multilingual children ages 3 to 13. Based on interviews and parental feedback, EMBO believes that parents did not bring their children to the conference because they may have been unsure about the program's suitability. Publishing the results of the pilot child care program and undertaking additional outreach will ensure that more researchers bring their children to EMBO 2010.

Sustainability: The EMBO child care pilot is considered a success by its organizers, serving as a highly visible experiment in creating a more family friendly academia. The EMBO program will be sustained and embedded in the 2010 EMBO conference and, perhaps, future conferences.

2009 AWARDS

Awardee: University of Massachusetts-Amherst

Project title: Family Travel Initiative.

Original goal: To promote and facilitate professional travel for STEM faculty and postdoctoral fellows with family responsibilities, one program encompassing the Five College system (UMass Amherst, Amherst, Hampshire, Smith, and Mount Holyoke colleges) will be developed. A second goal is to make the need for professional travel child care support "visible" and encourage future conference organizers to take responsibility for on-site child care as a policy objective.

Award period: Three years.

Accomplishments: The Five College system has proportionately more women scientists and engineers with children than any other universities (72% at the Five Colleges vs 42% nationally). The program aimed to educate early career STEM women about the critical importance of travel for professional advancement and to deliver biannual educational seminars, create postdoctorate/faculty travel-mentoring networks, dependent-care travel funding, and child care-support advocacy to professional societies and conference organizers. By the end of the project period, the STEM Family Travel Initiative (STEM-FTI) was smoothly conducting normal operations and exploring new avenues to increase its impact. Its interactive Web site (www.stemfamilytravel.org) describes the mission and includes applications for travel-support awards, announcements of educational programs, summaries of past workshops, updated listings of professional societies offering child care and how to access it, and a survey targeting national-level input on the level of interest in on-site child care at professional meetings of relatively large societies. Links to the STEM-FTI Web site from the Faculty Development and Human Resources Departments at each of the Five Colleges are in place, and links to/from professional societies to the Web site are increasing. Travel support was provided for 49 individuals across a broad group of disciplines, including life sciences, physical sciences, applied sciences, and engineering. Some support was for academics traveling to granting agencies for workshops and panels, an important component of academic networking often translating indirectly to research funding.

The education programs were extended beyond the Five College institutions to venues at the professional societies themselves, connecting with their advocacy mission. Free membership to a national, web-based babysitter bulletin board (SitterCity) has been provided by UMass to its faculty, while its fees were covered by travel grants to the faculty at the other Five Colleges. As a starting point for professional societies interested in pursuing on-site care, the program has also identified and contacted agencies that provide bonded child care at meetings and corporate events and maintain updated cost estimates for their services at technical meetings. Another strategy to mitigate the burden of finding reliable child care for academic travelers was to engage a formal nanny/babysitting network, i.e., a company that uses its own providers. As a result of these efforts, UMass has a contract with Parents in a Pinch for travelers and faculty in need of short-term dependent-care support in the Amherst area. Advocacy to professional societies is ongoing to raise awareness within the leadership of professional societies concerning the issues surrounding meeting travel and dependent care. STEM-FTI aims to plant the seeds for affordable child care at large meetings. First, as part of the travel-grant program, letters will be sent to contacts at professional societies sponsoring the conferences to which the grantees intend to travel.

Sustainability: STEM-FTI continues to meet its educational targets through holding formal workshops and other vehicles and providing monetary travel support to a diverse body of academics. Funds from the member centers have allowed continuation of operations beyond the originally funded period. SitterCity is now growing as a resource used for finding caregivers. The addition of Parents in a Pinch is proving sufficiently effective that the contract has been renewed and continued growth in the use of this new resource is evident.

The advocacy activities continue at the levels of the individual, professional society, agency, campus, and government. In 2012, STEM-FTI obtained a no-cost extension to continue beyond the formal end of its term (in early 2013) for an additional two years. The sustained presence of STEM-FTI will bolster its impact without requiring new resources. Toward a lasting impact, STEM-FTI initiated efforts starting in 2012 to forge connections to other institutions. Some of these efforts include joint presentations, including educational materials developed in collaboration with other institutions.

Awardee: University of California, Los Angeles

Project title: Enhancing the Academic Climate for STEM Women Scholars Through Family-Friendly Policies.

Original goal: To identify and confront family-related barriers, to encourage retention of women faculty by reducing the impact of workload following childbirth or adoption, and to increase entry of women into academic or research careers by facilitating opportunities for those with child care responsibilities to attend professional meetings.

Award period: Three years.

Accomplishments: The focus of the project was to help alleviate some of the stress associated with professional travel while caring for young children. All three elements of the project (policy, matching funds for maternity leave, and travel grants) comprised an integrative approach. Coupled with the quantitative and qualitative research already undertaken by University of California, Los Angeles (UCLA), a compelling model was developed for creating a more family friendly academy for UCLA and other large and diverse university systems across the United States. The program now consists of three parts: travel child care awards, matching-support funds for active service-modified duties (ASMD), and informational programs about family friendly policies and programs for female scholars in science, health, and engineering. The activities were promoted through the UCLA Faculty Diversity and Development Web site and direct e-mails to female postdoctoral scholars, assistant professors, and associate professors, as well as to deans, department chairs, and department administrators. The programs were also promoted in meetings with department chairs and orientations for new faculty members and new department chairs. Since 2010, 76 awards for travel child care were made, with eight divisions of the institution eligible: engineering, life sciences, physical sciences, public health, dentistry, medicine, nursing, and social sciences.

The active service-modified duties program deployed matching funds to assist-ladder rank women faculty members in science, health, and technology in using the university's ASMD policy. These funds were used to enable modified or reduced duties (e.g., teaching relief, departmental service, etc.) for one academic quarter, following the birth or adoption of a young child. This option was particularly significant for women faculty members in laboratory sciences, who often prefer a reduced schedule to taking off full time for a quarter due to the need to maintain research productivity. Providing matching-support funds to female faculty members and their departments facilitated this approach. In the three years of the program, 10 matching fund grants for active service-modified duties were made. The program also increased the dissemination of information about family friendly policies to academic women in science, health, and engineering, as well as to department chairs, deans, and all faculty members. A 12-page booklet, "Balancing Work and Life as an Assistant Professor," was developed, including sections on family friendly policies, time management, resources for child care, programs for children and families, managing service commitments and sleep, exercise, and a healthy diet. This booklet was well received and is now posted on the Faculty Diversity and Development Web site for convenient access.

Sustainability: Work continues on improving communication about family friendly policies and programs available at the university and the departmental climate for women and families. The interest in the Child Care Travel Grant Program has extended beyond the eligible departments and has become a model for other schools within UCLA. In 2011, both the UCLA School of Law and the Division of Humanities implemented their own Child Care Travel Grant programs, modeled after the original programs. The programs' success has grown over the years, due in part to deans and department chairs endorsing and helping to promote both the Travel Child Care Awards and the Active Service-Modified Duties programs by distributing information about them to faculty and postdoctoral scholars in their divisions/schools. In this way, awareness of the ASMD program has increased among deans and department chairs as well, fulfilling one of the goals of the project. During 2013, an ongoing Travel Child Care Award program will be created, with funding provided by the deans of UCLA's schools and divisions, thereby institutionalizing this much-needed assistance for women in the early stages of their academic careers.

Awardee: University of Groningen

Project title: Special Child Care Program at the University of Groningen.

Original goal: To implement a new child care program that complements the standard daycare program for ad hoc situations (a sick child, travel to conferences, and parental participation in international projects); child care for guest lecturers; and care for the children of visiting participants at conferences organized by the university.

Award period: Two years.

Accomplishments: The University of Groningen is addressing a growing issue in the Netherlands in a pragmatic way. The percentage of women professors at the university, at 14%, is only slightly higher than the Dutch average. While there are currently daytime care facilities for children at the university, definite gaps exist in helping women scholars further increase their professional participation and travel, ultimately leading to improved academic career development and viability. This project represents a very basic child care program without advocacy, mentoring, or work/life balance components, though those elements may be incorporated into the program in future years. The child care program was successfully implemented for temporary guest lecturers and guest researchers and for participants at conferences organized by the university. However, complications have arisen in developing a program for child care in ad hoc situations (such as illness of a child, conference attendance of the parent, or parent participation in a collaborative project abroad). Efforts in year two focused on developing a program that can cover such situations with the most flexibility and in the context of the strict legal requirements covering daycare centers and sick children.

Sustainability: There is currently no other university within the Netherlands that provides this kind of child care program. It has the potential to serve as a recruitment draw and a model for other universities and institutes within the Netherlands and Europe at large. If the program is successful, the university has pledged support after the funding period has elapsed.

Awardee: Third World Organization for Women in Science

Project title: Women Scientists in the Developing World Awards.

Original goal: To enhance the role of women scientists and technologists in the developing world and to increase the international visibility of research being conducted by young women scientists working and living in developing countries by increasing the number of awards available.

Award period: Two years.

Accomplishments: To address the less than 10% success rate of young women scientists from developing countries in the Young Scientists Awards program of The Academy of Sciences for the Developing World (TWAS), the Third World Organization for Women in Science (TWOWS) launched a new program of awards to highlight the work of excellent young women scientists from developing countries. Additional support from the Elsevier Foundation permitted the expansion of the program to offer individual awards of $5000 to a larger number of young women scientists. More than 600 women from 55 countries attended the TWOWS conference in June 2010 in Beijing, at which 12 awards were given to outstanding young women scientists: one each in biology, chemistry and physics/mathematics from each of the four regions recognized by TWOWS: Asia, Middle East, sub-Saharan Africa, and Latin America. The award program will continue in 2011 under the auspices of the Organization for Women Scientists for the Developing World (OWSDW), the new name TWOWS adopted in Beijing.

Sustainability: TWOWS anticipates that the program can be sustained and expanded by its seeking additional funds from donor agencies.

2010 AWARDS

Awardee: Organization for Women in Science for the Developing World

Project title: National Assessments and Benchmarking of Gender, Science, Technology and Innovation: Gender Equality and Innovation Society (GEIS) Framework.

Original goal: To chart policies, factors, and key elements for a global view on the participation of women scientists and technologists across seven countries (China, India, Brazil, Indonesia, South Africa, the United States, and Europe).

Award period: One year.

Accomplishments: OWSDW has formalized its processes and procedures for data analysis and benchmarking. A collaborative arrangement with the University of Maryland Center for International Digital Governance will provide capabilities in longitudinal and correlative data analysis for the indicators previously identified in the GEIS framework. That data analysis software also will support intra- and intercountry comparisons. To generate data for the benchmarking and forecasting software program (FutureInnovate), knowledgeable respondents at the national level in the chosen countries will be queried on the participation of women in their science and technology enterprise. These surveys will also test the viability of such data collection in these countries. The current countries for study are Brazil, South Korea, the European Union, the United States, and possibly Indonesia, or Malaysia. Unfortunately, China declined to be a part of the study at this time and OWSDW moved forward without their participation after extensive consultation with Elsevier Foundation leadership and China experts. The timing of the national studies will be staggered, starting with Brazil and South Korea, where researchers with extensive experience in policy analysis and data collection will initiate work and be prepared to make adjustments and pass on lessons learned to those countries "coming online" later in the study. The United States and European Union will comprise the next phase, with other countries added as experience is gained in implementation of the data collection and analysis.

Sustainability: It is anticipated that the basis and approaches for collecting and assessing data will provide not only significant information about the countries currently under study, but also important context for potential expansion to a broader array of countries in future years.

Awardee: Organization for Women for Science in the Developing World

Project title: OWSD Women Scientists in the Developing World Awards.

Original goal: To support 12 regional and discipline-specific prizes for young women scientists in each of the four regions of the developing world (Africa, Latin America, the Caribbean, and the Middle East) for a total of three prizes per region in biological sciences, chemical sciences, and the physical and mathematical sciences.

Award period: One year.

Accomplishments/Sustainability: The expanded prizes will ensure that talented young women scientists in developing countries are recognized for excellence within their own disciplines and will help to promote the overall participation and recognition of women scientists in the developing world.

2011 AWARDS

Awardee: Association for Women in Science

Project title: Rethinking the Future of the STEM Workforce: Best Practices in Work/life Effectiveness.

Original goal: While women comprise roughly half the US workforce, they hold just 24% of STEM jobs, according to the Department of Commerce. Whether the root causes lie in a lack of female role models, gender stereotyping, or a lack of family friendly workplace flexibility, the resulting attrition in the academic pipeline means that the United States is halving its potential for innovation. The objectives of this project are to: (1) distill and leverage best practices and internationally transportable strategies in support of institutional change to accommodate work/life in STEM employment; (2) create a best-practices report that could serve as an action plan to help STEM employers, policy makers, and working women identify and create systemic change; and (3) enhance visibility for the Elsevier Foundation and AWIS as thought leaders in attainment of work/life effectiveness in the STEM disciplines. AWIS will collaborate with the New Scholars program to leverage best practice testimony to impel systemic change in the global STEM workplace.

Project period: Two years.

Accomplishments: To inform the proposed dialogue, a survey of work/life options, access, and usage in the global STEM workplace was conducted in late 2011 by Elsevier's research arm. Through an international work/life satisfaction survey and a New Scholars Roundtable, AWIS distilled recommendations into a report that will serve as an action plan to help employers, working women, and policy makers identify, create, and sustain systemic changes in the workplace. The survey provided a snapshot of both men's and women's perspectives on and practices around work/life issues, including workplace flexibility, family-responsive policies, and dual-career challenges. Survey results were distributed and discussed at a convening of global experts in New York City in March 2012, at which AWIS convened 20 of the most successful New Scholars Program representatives and other global experts in work/life, STEM employment best practices, and workplace change. Informed by the survey outcomes, the goals of this global "think tank" included: an understanding of the emerging and pressing concerns of today's Global STEM workforce regarding work/life and the advancement of working women; capturing recommendations from thought leaders and practitioners who are leading efforts in work/life effectiveness, diversity, and workplace equity about the tools, resources, and policy changes needed; and distilling the recommendations into a report that would serve as an action plan to help employers, working women, and policy makers identify, create, and sustain systemic changes.

Sustainability: The key findings of the project will be compiled into a book covering the following concepts: work/life issues through the international survey results: dual careers and strategic decision making; work/life issues; child care/dependent care in professional contexts, promoting family friendly policies, the effect of implicit bias on the workplace and how it effects work/life choices; mentoring and networking; and future directions in United States federal grant policy for child care. Resources, workshops, presentations, and outreach will be made to large numbers of influencers across disciplines and sectors through the AWIS Web site, chapters, and partners, including scientific societies. The overall goal of the publication is to increase the visibility for both the Elsevier Foundation and AWIS as STEM thought leaders in work/life effectiveness.

Awardee: Portia Ltd

Project title: Scenario Toolkit for Advancing Careers in Science.

Original goal: To help individuals, and women in particular, to navigate more effectively the complex array of relationships between events and decision points that shape a scientist's professional development and career path. The project aims to use the participatory method of scenario construction as a tool to enable science institutions to support their early career researchers (in particular, women) in making more informed and effective professional- and personal-development decisions focused on career related issues. "Creating Futures in Science," as the workshops are called, represents a holistic approach, combining reflection, homework, and a program of activities to show the young researchers what kind of options they have; how the research system works; where to find the right role models; how to avoid cultural stereotypes, and managing family life. Career issues and environments are viewed at the micro (personal and within an institution) and macro (national, cross-sector, international) levels.

Award period: Three years.

Accomplishments: The project uses the Scenario Method, which is well understood and has been widely tested, although not in the context proposed here. Traditionally, the Scenario Method has been used in social-policy settings to help direct attention to driving forces, possible avenues of change, and the span of contingencies that may be confronted. Here, the method will be adapted to focus on events and decision points that influence the direction and progress of an individual's science career. The group-based and participatory nature of the Scenario Method promotes sharing of knowledge and experience, peer learning, and team spirit and collaboration when identifying and analyzing career choices and pathways, dominant future-oriented trends, events that can alter the future environment, and the roles of stakeholders. The method offers institutions a way to overcome two common gender problems: (1) how to recruit women into fields in which they are in a minority and thus where sufficient role models are not available to act as examples or mentors, by engaging potential applicants to enroll in university courses in participatory exploration of the career landscape, and (2) how to advance women already in the system to higher levels by helping them increase the number of applications for key research grants awards, and inclusion in nominations to important leadership roles and decision-making committees and panels.

During the first year, two pilot workshops were held in two very different environments: Fraunhofer Gesellschaft in Berlin and Tel Aviv University. Both partners have extensive experience and expertise in the areas of gender, academic careers, mentoring, facilitation, and participatory methods. This knowledge ensured effective collaboration and intellectually productive analysis of the work and outputs at each stage. The project concept was presented at a conference on gender and higher education in Bergen, Norway in August and at the 2012 European Gender Summit. Both workshops were highly rated and oversubscribed despite significant differences in participant profiles, academic interests, institutional cultures, and social traditions. As a result of the experience gained in the workshops, Portia Ltd identified a research gap in how men and women scientists construct the role of the family and work/life balance in their career decision-making processes. Women in both societies grapple with conflicting societal forces (approval of women's pursuit of higher education coupled with an equally strong expectation of a woman's full commitment to family life). Further research into these issues could help early career researchers (and their mentors) navigate these issues more effectively.

Sustainability: Portia Ltd is now testing how adaptable the workshop is to different academic cultures. ETH Zurich, one of the top research universities in Europe, has invited the project partners to perform the Berlin workshop there in 2013. As ETH is a member of the League of European Research Universities (LERU, with over 21 members), a successful workshop at ETH will help promote the program to the other members given the strong fit with LERU's strategic commitment to gender equality. In addition to running pilot workshops during the second year, the project will also prepare for a stakeholder-evaluation workshop and promotion of the method and project through Portia's contact database of more than 7500 international individuals and scientific organizations. The 2013 Gender Summit will take place in Washington, DC, providing an important reporting opportunity to reach a United States audience.

Awardee: University of Nebraska-Lincoln

Project title: STEM Committee on Institutional Cooperation (CIC) Writing Retreat.

Original goal: The project goal is to develop, pilot, and evaluate the retention of women scientists by improving research productivity and promoting critical networks. The writing retreat is a well-established method used extensively in the humanities to stimulate productivity, networks, and confidence, but has not been as widely used in STEM fields. A week long, multidisciplinary, multirank writing retreat at the University of Nebraska, Lincoln conference was offered to STEM faculty across the "Big 10" universities.

Award period: Two years.

Accomplishments: The writing retreat was held in June 2012 and was built on the analysis of a writing retreat for women geoscientists at UNL, providing proof-of-concept that scientists' productivity and work/life satisfaction both increase post retreat. The STEM retreat expanded the concept across disciplines and universities, reaching out to Big 10 or CIC institutions that already have a longstanding tradition of collaborative research, library resources, and regular meetings among deans, department chairs, and heads of member institutions. The inclusion of a special child care program, a partnership with the Lincoln Children's Museum, enabled faculty to bring their children for a science day camp during the retreat and have in depth discussions with fellow scientist parents on work/life integration. Normalizing family accommodations has been shown to be critical to enabling new STEM scholars' greater involvement and participation in writing retreats, conferences, and organizational meetings. The STEM retreat supported 21 faculty members, 12 of whom brought children, from a range of disciplines including medicine, anthropology, zoology, chemistry, statistics, environment, bio molecular engineering, civil engineering, geography, sociology, limnology, and atmospheric sciences. They were drawn from the Universities of Chicago, Wisconsin, and Nebraska; Florida State, Purdue, and Michigan State universities; and also non-Big 10 universities. Professional writing coaching and peer feedback were mixed with large blocks of unstructured writing time to improve writing success, plus work/life balance discussions, and communal meals.

Sustainability: As a follow up, quarterly writing "accountability and support" webinars have been offered on scholarly publishing, the tenure process, leadership, and issues related to increasing retention of women in academia in STEM fields. One positive retreat outcome has been the writing groups started by many academics when they returned to their home institutions. Many of the participants have also reported greatly improved writing habits post retreat and are statistically more likely to report that they have developed a structured writing schedule. During the evaluation phase, the UNL team will compare different types of writing retreats (in person, in person with videoconference, a single vs multidisciplinary or multiinstitutional approach) to isolate the most important ingredient for facilitating success. Their analysis will be finalized after participants complete a 12-month posttest survey and are compared with peers from their department who did not attend the retreat. The overall project will result in a concise best-practice guide to cost-effective, targeted STEM writing retreats.

Awardee: University of Carthage, Engineering School of Communications, Tunisia

Project title: Get Ahead with Optics: Career Development for Women in Science.

Original goal: Over the last few years, optics research has become an indispensable part of daily life. Fiber optics for telecommunications, medical imaging, cancer research, optical parts in automobiles, and computer and 3D screens are at the core of the world's technical infrastructure. This interdisciplinary proposal had as its goal to orient young women scientists in the dynamic and rapidly evolving field of optics and photonics while providing them with professional-development skills and a deeper understanding of what is needed to succeed as a woman scientist.

Award period: One year.

Accomplishments: The project scope noted that, with women as 50% of all customers and users of technological products, the economy needs more women designers to create innovative products closer to women's needs. The 10-day "summer school" in optics in September 2012 was a partnership between the University of Carthage's Engineering School of Communications and Philipps University of Marburg, Germany. Recent Tunisian and German PhD graduates (26 participants) were provided with scientific orientation, career coaching, and international networking to lay the groundwork for a successful scientific career. The project occurred at a turning point for both the young women researchers and Tunisia as an emerging democracy and role model of the Arab Spring. One of the goals of the Optics Summer School was to enable a country with few advanced training programs for women to create a compelling model for future collaborations across other disciplines. The scientific portion of the program included classes on fluorescence, tissue optics, new optical markers, spectroscopy, microscopy, breast cancer imaging, laser application, optical signal processing, fiber optics, Matlab and statistic, photonics, crystal fibers and applications, and nanophotonics. The professional development courses focused on postgraduation skills including writing a scientific paper, use of End Note, presentation skills, job interview skills, project and time management, leadership style, conflict management, and body language. The summer school also focused on succeeding as a woman scientist in a male-dominated academic field. Evening discussion sessions covered work/life balance, networking, industry vs academia career choices, and managing conflicts with male colleagues. Three high-profile keynote women scientists were invited to be keynote speakers and to provide perspective on research careers in optics and navigating the academic pipeline.

Sustainability: The evaluation of the summer school was extremely positive and the organizers are keen to expand the concept to include 50 international students, student presentations, and an annual career-development meeting.

2012 AWARDS

Awardee: Appalachian State University

Project title: The Appalachian Women Scientists Program.

Original goal: Women scientists often choose to work at smaller institutions because they consider these institutions more family friendly. According to a report from the University of California-Berkeley and the Center for American Progress, women scholars report that they consider research-intensive universities the least family friendly career choice, with fewer than half (43%) of highly trained women scientists at US universities working at major research institutions. Most female doctorate holders in science and engineering work at smaller institutions, with 19% at master's-granting institutions like Appalachian State University. Targeting a midsized public university in rural North Carolina, the Appalachian Women Scientists programs aim to establish an affordable national model enabling smaller institutions to support women scientists' professional development.

Award period: Two years.

Accomplishments (anticipated): The project will provide direct financial support for professional travel and dependent-care expenses so that scientists can engage in activities essential to their research careers, regardless of their family obligations. This support will be provided through informational and social support via workshops, web content, and mentoring to help faculty balance work/life responsibilities and connect faculty with other local and university resources for professional women and parents. It will also include seed grants to encourage interinstitutional research collaboration; educate academic administrators and campus leadership about the challenges facing women scientists; and, finally, use data gathered from this project to advocate for family-responsive policies. The inclusion of male scientists, who also face many of the same challenges, will be a facet of the program.

Sustainability: The project should demonstrate ways in which the careers of female (and male) scientists in small-scale, isolated settings can be strategically promoted. Scientists who choose to work at smaller institutions face different challenges in building their research careers. While they may enjoy better work/life balance, they also have heavier teaching loads, lower salaries, less internal funding for professional travel and early career research, and less well-equipped on-campus research laboratories and computing and administrative infrastructure. In addition, institutions with fewer faculty members also offer fewer mentors and role models for women scientists, fewer potential collaborators for scientists in highly-specialized fields, and less peer support for early-career scientists who may be the only women (and/or mothers) within their departments. By providing low-cost financial, mentoring, and social support for these women scientists and documenting the return on investment in terms of promotion, tenure attainment, retention, and research productivity, the Appalachian Women Scientists program should be able to demonstrate that women scientists can choose to work at a smaller institution for work/life balance reasons without stunting their research careers.

Awardee: National Postdoctoral Association

Project title: The National Postdoc-Societies Collaboration to Boost Retention of Women Scientists.

Original goal: The postdoctoral training period has a significant impact upon science, health, and society at national and international levels. It represents a critical transition point in the academic pipeline at which the number of women scientists and engineers declines significantly. While the relative number of women decreases at every step along a research-career path, the heaviest attrition occurs before tenure track and in the fields with the largest numbers of postdocs. Increasingly, the postdoctoral position has become required for advancement, creating an additional career step and lengthening the total time until the first permanent position is attained. Also, the likelihood that a postdoc will obtain a tenure-track position has decreased significantly. However, the factors that most strongly influence the career decisions of postdoc women are related to family formation, isolation, and low self-confidence resulting from lack of mentoring and encouragement. This proposal, from an organization experienced in addressing the quality of the postdoc experience, will tackle this loss of talent through a targeted collaboration with scientific societies to produce a postdoc guidebook for navigating the academic pipeline.

Award period: Two years.

Accomplishments (anticipated): Through focus groups, the National Postdoctoral Association (NPA) has identified the key providers of professional development for postdoc women: their mentors, institutions, and professional societies. This proposal aims to expand the role of professional societies and has identified more than 200 multidisciplinary associations to participate in this effort. Currently, the majority of professional postdoc development opportunities focus on biomedicine, which represents the largest postdoc population at most institutions. Nonbiomedical postdocs in the focus groups believed that there were very few relevant opportunities offered to them. The NPA's multidisciplinary society collaboration should help address this imbalance by identifying both the discipline-specific needs of postdoc women and the necessary resources. Key NPA project activities will include surveying societies and associations, conducting focus groups at the NPA 2013 Annual Meeting, adapting the practices identified, creating an online clearinghouse to disseminate these practices, and developing a society workshop track at the 2014 NPA Annual Conference to define and disseminate best practices.

Sustainability: A postdoc workshop model will be developed that can be easily implemented across annual society meetings. Publication and dissemination of the new postdoc resource guide will also have the potential of serving as a catalyst for the scientific societies not yet addressing postdoc attrition issues.

Awardee: Academy of Sciences for the Developing World (TWAS)/Organization for Women for Science in the Developing World

Project title: The Elsevier Foundation Awards for Early Career Women Scientists in the Developing World.

Original goal: The Elsevier Foundation has committed to supporting the recognition for women scientists in the developing world. These awards serve to highlight the importance of women researchers in emerging countries, and to provide valuable international recognition for scientists in the developing world.

Award period: Three years.

Accomplishments (anticipated): The awards program builds on the previous awards in 2009 to the TWOWS and in 2010 to the OWSD, but now provides a deeper focus on discipline and professional visibility. It also represents a more explicit partnership with the TWAS on the part of the Elsevier Foundation. The five region-specific annual prizes will rotate between life sciences in 2013 and chemistry and physics/math in the subsequent two years. Nominations will be accepted from early career scientists (within 10 years of graduating with a PhD degree) from the 81 countries with low scientific output as defined by TWAS. They will be reviewed by a committee of distinguished life scientists chaired by the OWSD president. Award winners will receive their awards at the annual American Association for the Advancement of Science meeting.

Sustainability: Funding for awards through the Elsevier Foundation is in place through 2015.

Awardee: Women in Global Science and Technology

Project title: National Assessments in Gender and Science, Technology and Innovation (STI) in Latin America.

Original goal: This project builds on a previous Elsevier Foundation grant in 2010 to Women in Global Science and Technology (WISAT) and the OWSDW, supporting the assessment of five countries with highly accelerated growth in the research arena: South Korea, India, Brazil, Indonesia, and South Africa. The WISAT follow-up proposal calls for an expansion of the National Assessments from 9 to 11 more countries. It aims to build on Phase 1 findings and country analyses by expanding to Argentina, Chile, and Mexico (Latin America). Future assessments are anticipated for Kuwait, United Arab Emirates (Arab States); Ghana and Senegal (Africa); and Pakistan and Thailand (pending identification of appropriate partners). Countries are chosen on the basis of their knowledge economy and the state of their STI system (including policy, education and innovation capacity); and potential for data collection and analysis.

Award period: One year.

Accomplishments: In the previous grant award, existing qualitative and quantitative research from the United States and European Union were compared and analyzed to map the opportunities and obstacles faced by women in these countries. The results yielded significant media coverage and interest from policy makers as they build programs to improve status, shift policy, and develop new projects based on real data and statistics. The Gender Equality Knowledge Society (GEKS) indicator framework was developed to address the situation in which women, particularly in the developing world, continue to be on the wrong side of the digital and innovation divides. Women generally experience lower levels of access to information and technology, and are poorly represented in education, entrepreneurship, and employment in STI fields. Gaps in women's access to resources, opportunities, rights, education, and financing greatly diminish the potential of a country to achieve progress, reduce poverty, and improve the overall quality of life.

Current STI indexes do not include gender equality issues, nor do the global gender equality indexes address STI. The innovative GEKS framework highlights the interrelations between them and looks at the ability of women and men to participate in STI: access to science and technology education, access to and use of technology, decision making in knowledge-society sectors, participation in science, technology, and innovation systems, and access to lifelong learning. It then assesses the base conditions for socioeconomic and political development that determine the ability of both women and men to contribute to the knowledge society: health status, social and economic status, type of opportunities available, level of political participation, access to resources, and policy environment. In this new award, WISAT will focus on assessments in Argentina, Chile, and Mexico.

Sustainability: This project is expected to continue the demonstration of an analytical approach to gender assessments. The results should continue to inform not only policy makers and other stakeholders in their work to promote women in STI in the countries involved, but also academic researchers on women in science and technology globally. It is anticipated that this approach will stimulate interest on the part of other funding entities. For example, the original Elsevier Foundation funding in 2009 provided a valuable proof-of-concept and led to a Swedish Development Agency grant to support four studies in four countries in East Africa (Kenya, Rwanda, Tanzania, and Uganda) in 2012–2013.

Appendix C. Researcher Insights Survey Questions for Data Collection

Indicate how strongly you agree or disagree with the following statements:

1. Discovery (i.e., expanding knowledge) is the main reason why I undertake research.
2. I feel like the work I am doing is making a difference to the society.
3. I am satisfied with my career opportunities.
4. I am happy with my work/life balance (e.g., time spent working vs time spent on my personal life).
5. I am comfortable saying no to work/projects that I do not consider a priority.
6. At work there are others to whom I can delegate tasks.
7. Ensuring I have good work/life balance has negatively impacted my career.
8. There is sufficient support for my partner/spouse at my institution.
9. I have delayed having children in order to pursue my career in research.
10. I am considering moving to another country to further my career in research.

Please respond to the following questions:

11. What has been your attitude toward stress at work?
12. How often do work demands conflict with life demands?
13. On average, approximately how many hours do you work per week?
14. How do you feel about your current position?
15. If you expect to leave your current role, please identify the major reasons why you wish to leave.

References

1. Sprunt E, Howes S. Results of dual-career couple survey. *J Pet Tech* 2011;**63**(10):60–2.
2. Sprunt E, Howes S. Dual career couple survey results. Paper SPE 151971-MS. One Petro. Available from: http://www.onepetro.org/mslib/app/Preview.do?paperNumber=SPE-151971-MS&societyCode=SPE; 2011.
3. Sprunt E, Howes S. Factors impacting dual-career couples. Results of December 2011 talent council survey. Paper SPE 160928-MS. One Petro. Available from: http://www.onepetro.org/mslib/app/Preview.do?paperNumber=SPE-160928-MS&societyCode=SPE; 2012.
4. awis.org [Internet]. Alexandria (VA): Association for Women in Science. Available from: http://www.awis.org/associations/9417/files/AWIS_Work_Life_Balance_Executive_Summary.pdf; [March 8, 2012; accessed 09.08.13].
5. info.sciverse.com [Internet]. Amsterdam: Elsevier BV; c2013. Available from: http://www.info.sciverse.com/scopus; [March 8, 2012; accessed 09.08.13].
6. Committee on Maximizing the Potential of Women in Academic Science and Engineering, National Academy of Sciences, National Academy of Engineering, and Institute of Medicine. *Beyond bias and barriers: fulfilling the potential of women in academic science and engineering*. Washington (DC): The National Academies Press; 2007. Available from: http://www.nap.edu/catalog.php?record_id=11741.
7. Monosson E, editor. *Motherhood: the elephant in the laboratory-women scientists speak out*. Ithaca (NY): Cornell University Press; 2008.
8. www.nsf.gov [Internet]. Arlington (VA): National Science Foundation; Science and Engineering Indicators 2008. Available from: http://www.nsf.gov/statistics/seind08/; [March 8, 2012; accessed 09.08.13].
9. Pritchard PA, editor. *Success strategies for women in science: a portable mentor*. Burlington (MA): Academic Press; 2006.
10. mccu.ge [Internet]. Tbilisi (GE): Maternal and Child Care Union; c2012. Available from: www.mccu.ge/elsevier.htm; [March 8, 2012; accessed 09.08.13].
11. advance.unl.edu [Internet]. Lincoln (NE): ADVANCE-Nebraska, University of Nebraska, Lincoln; c2013. Available from: http://advance.unl.edu/; [March 8, 2012; accessed 09.08.13].
12. wesleyan.edu/gain/workshops/assessment.html [Internet]. Middletown (CT): Geoscience Academics in the Northeast, GAIN; [March 8, 2012; accessed 09.08.13].
13. Holmes MA, O'Connell S. Women geoscientists' writing retreat. *AWIS Magazine* 2007;**36**(4):22–3.
14. O'Connell S, Holmes MA. Retreating to advance women geoscience faculty. *EOS Trans Am Geophys Union* 2007;**88**(47).
15. advance.unl.edu [Internet]. Lincoln (NE): ADVANCE-Nebraska STEM Writing Retreat, University of Nebraska, Lincoln; c2013. Available from: advance.unl.edu/big-ten-stem-writing-retreat; [March 8, 2012; accessed 09.08.13].
16. Hill, PW. UNL's big TEN STEM writing retreat a success! [Internet]. Lincoln (NE). Available from: http://advance.unl.edu/newsletters/Enewsv4No2August172012.pdf; [March 8, 2012; accessed 09.08.13].
17. atlasvanlines.com [Internet]. Evansville (IN): Atlas Van Lines, Inc.; c2011. Corporate Relocation Survey 2011. Available from: http://www.atlasvanlines.com/relocation-surveys/corporate-relocation/2011/; [accessed 09.08.13].

18. compensationforce.com [Internet]. Olathe (KS): Compdata Surveys; c2011 and c2013. Compensation Force BenchmarkProSurveys, 2012 Voluntary Turnover Rates by Industry. Available from: http://www.compensationforce.com/miscellaneous/; [March 8, 2012; accessed 09.08.13].

19. Minton-Eversole T. Easing the travails of trailing spouses. *HR Magazine* November 1, 2011;**56**(11). Available from: http://www.shrm.org/Publications/hrmagazine/EditorialContent/2011/1111/Pages/1111eversole.aspx.

20. hirecentrix.com [Internet]. San Diego: HireCentrix, Inc.; c2010. Available from: http://www.hirecentrix.com/cost-of-employee-turnover.html; [March 8, 2012; accessed 09.08.13].

21. webpronews.com [Internet]. Lexington (KY): c1998–2013. Available from: http://www.webpronews.com/employee-retention-what-employee-turnover-really-costs-your-company-2006-07; [March 8, 2012; accessed 09.08.13].

22. Schiebinger L, Henderson AD, Gilmartin SK. Dual career academic couples: what universities need to know. Stanford University [Internet]; August, 2008. Available from: http://gender.stanford.edu/sites/default/files/DualCareerFinal_0.pdf; [March 8, 2012; accessed 09.08.13].

23. techvalleyconnect.org [Internet]. Troy (NY): Tech Valley Connect; c2013. Available from: http://www.techvalleyconnect.org/; [accessed 09.08.13].

24. portiaweb.org.uk [Internet]. London; c2013. Available from: http://www.portiaweb.org.uk/index.php/2012-07-11-23-46-44/creating-futures-in-science; [accessed 09.08.13].

25. Whittington KB. Mothers of invention? Gender, motherhood, and new dimensions of productivity in the science profession. *Work Occup* 2011;**38**(3):417–56. Available from: http://academic.reed.edu/sociology/faculty/whittington/docs/Whittington_WorkandOccupations_2011.pdf.

26. curt-rice.com [Internet]. Tromso; c2013. How to get more women professors: success on the top of the world! Available from: http://curt-rice.com/2011/12/03/how-to-get-more-women-professors-success-on-the-top-of-the-world/; [March 8, 2012; accessed 09.08.13].

27. daphnejackson.org [Internet]. Surrey (UK): The Daphne Jackson Trust. Daphne Jackson Fellowships for Women Returners. Available from: http://www.daphnejackson.org; [March 8, 2012; accessed 09.08.13].

28. Sjoberg O. Ambivalent attitudes, contradictory institutions. Ambivalence in gender-role attitudes in comparative perspective. *Int J Comp Sociol* 2010;**51**(1–2):33–57.

29. Kaplan KA. Dual dilemma. *Nature* 2010;**466**:1144–5. Available from: http://www.nature.com/naturejobs/2010/100826/full/nj7310-1144a.html.

30. Byrnes J, Miller DC, Schafer WD. Gender differences in risk taking: a meta-analysis. *Psychol Bull* 1999;**125**:367–83.

31. Xie Y. Social influences on science and engineering career decisions. National Academy of Sciences (US), National Academy of Engineering (US), and Institute of Medicine (US) Committee on Maximizing the Potential of Women in Academic Science and Engineering Biological, social, and organizational components of success for women in academic science and engineering. Washington (DC): National Academies Press (US); 2006. Available from: http://www.ncbi.nlm.nih.gov/books/NBK23777/.

32. erc.europa.eu. [Internet]. Brussels: What about a gender-equality plan in the ERC evaluation process, and is maternity leave part of the eligibility period? Available from: http://erc.europa.eu/faq/what-about-gender-equality-plan-erc-evaluation-process-and-maternity-leave-part-eligibility-peri; [March 8, 2012; accessed 09.08.13].

33. Risberg G, Johansson EE, Hamberg K. A theoretical model for analysing gender bias in medicine. *Int J Equity Health* 2009;**8**(28). Available from: http://www.equityhealthj.com/content/8/1/28.

34. eurodoc.net [Internet]. Brussels: European Council of Doctoral Candidates and Junior Researchers. The first Eurodoc survey on doctoral candidates in twelve European countries. Available from: http://www.eurodoc.net/projects/completed-projects/eurodoc-survey-i/; [March 8, 2012; accessed 09.08.13].

35. cpp.amu.edu.pl. [Internet]. Poznan. Center for Public Policy. EUROAC project on the academic profession in Europe: Response to societal change; c2006–2013. Available from: http://www.cpp.amu.edu.pl/euroac.htm; [March 8, 2012; accessed 09.08.13].

36. Laudel G, Gläser J. From apprentice to colleague. The metamorphosis of early career researchers. *High Educ* 2008;**55**:387–406. Available from: http://www.laudel.info/pdf/journal%20articles/08%20from%20apprentice.pdf.

37. Mason MA, Goulden M. Do babies matter? The effect of family formation on the life-long careers of academic men and women. *Academe* 2002;**88**(6):21–7. Available from: http://www.aas.org/cswa/status/2004/JANUARY2004/DoBabiesMatter.html.

38. academia-net.de [Internet]. Heidelberg: Robert Bosch Foundation; c2013. Available from: http://www.academia-net.de/; [March 8, 2012; accessed 09.08.13].

39. genderinscience.org [Internet]. London: genSET; c2013. Available from: http://www.genderinscience.org; [March 8, 2012; accessed 09.08.13].

40. http://gender-summit.eu [Internet]. London; c2013. Available from: http://www.gender-summit.eu; [March 8, 2012; accessed 09.08.13].

41. Ledin A, Bornmann L, Gannon F, Wallon G. A persistent problem. Traditional gender roles hold back female scientists. *EMBO Rep* 2007;**8**(11). Available from: http://www.embo.org/documents/WIS_report_2007_persistent_problem.pdf.

42. embo.org [Internet]. Heidelberg: European Molecular Biology Organization; c2013. Available from: http://www.the-embo-meeting.org/; [March 8, 2012; accessed 09.08.13].

43. Cox A. Under the microscope: EMBO initiatives. *Biochemist* October, 2009:48–9. Available from: http://www.biochemist.org/bio/03105/0048/031050048.pdf.

44. aps.org [Internet]. College Park (MD): American Physical Society Committee on the Status of Women in Physics CSWP Gazette 2009 Spring, Fall, 2010 Fall; c1981–2013. Available from: http://www.aps.org/programs/women/reports/gazette/index.cfm; [March 8, 2012; accessed 09.08.13].

45. Kaplan K. Grants aim to help women. *Nature* 2009;**458**(7242):1207.

46. Watt FM. Women in cell biology: getting to the top. *Nat Rev Mol Cell Biol* April, 2006;**7**:287–90.

47. ascb.org. [Internet]. Bethesda (MD): American Society for Cell Biology; c2013. Available from: http://am.ascb.org/meetings/index.php/travelchildcare-awards; [March 8, 2012; accessed 09.08.13].

48. Masur S, Nathke I, Roecklein-Canfield J, Weisz O. We've made it easier for ASCB members who are parents to attend the annual meeting. *ASCB Newsletter* 2013 August 10–11. Available from: http://am.ascb.org/newsletters/2013/August_NL/index.html#10.

49. stemfamilytravel.org [Internet]. Amherst (MA): STEM Family Travel Initiative. Available from: http://www.stemfamilytravel.org; [March 8, 2012; accessed 09.08.13].

50. nih.gov [Internet]. Bethesda (MD): National Institutes of Health. Conference Grants. Available from: http://grants.nih.gov/grants/funding/r13/r13_faqs.htm#570; [March 8, 2012; accessed 09.08.13].

51. stemfamilytravel.org. [Internet]. Amherst (MA): The role of travel in professional advancement. STEM Family Travel Initiative Educational Seminars. Available from: http://stemfamilytravel.org/facts/; [March 8, 2012; accessed 09.08.13].

52. stemfamilytravel.org [Internet]. Amherst (MA): Open letter for professional societies. STEM Family Travel Initiative Professional Society Advocacy. Available from: http://stemfamilytravel.org/wp-content/uploads/2010/03/OpenLetter.pdf; [March 8, 2012; accessed 09.08.13].

53. regulations.gov [Internet]. Washington (DC): Office of Management and Budget. Reform of federal policies relating to grants and cooperative agreements: cost principles and administrative requirements. Section 621 of proposed OMB Uniform Guidance: Cost Principles, audit, and administrative requirements for federal awards. Available from: http://www.regulations.gov/#!documentDetail;D=OMB-2013-0001-0001; [accessed 09.08.13].

54. faculty.diversity.ucla.edu [Internet]. Los Angeles: University of California Los Angeles Office of Faculty Diversity and Development, active service modified duties policy. Available from: https://faculty.diversity.ucla.edu/funding-opportunities-n/family-friendly-grants/benefits-and-privileges-of-apm-760; [March 8, 2012; accessed 09.08.13].

55. faculty.diversity.ucla.edu [Internet]. Los Angeles: UCLA family friendly grant program. Available from: https://faculty.diversity.ucla.edu/funding-opportunities-n/family-friendly-grants; [March 8, 2012; accessed 09.08.13].

56. faculty.diversity.ucla.edu [Internet]. Los Angeles: UCLA Faculty Diversity Family Friendly Academy. Available from: https://faculty.diversity.ucla.edu/resources-for/work-life/family-friendly-academy; [March 8, 2012; accessed 09.08.13].

57. faculty.diversity.ucla.edu [Internet]. Los Angeles: UCLA Faculty Diversity Resources. Balancing work and life as an assistant professor. Available from: https://faculty.diversity.ucla.edu/resources-for/work-life/family-friendly-academy/balancing-work-and-life-as-an-assistant-professor; [March 8, 2012; accessed 09.08.13].

58. princeton.edu [Internet]. Princeton (NJ); Princeton University; Benefits information and campus housing resources. Available from: http://www.princeton.edu/dof/professionals/ben_info/; [March 8, 2012; accessed 09.08.13].

59. princeton.edu [Internet]. Princeton (NJ); Princeton University; Numbered memoranda. Available from: http://www.princeton.edu/dof/policies/memos/; [March 8, 2012; accessed 09.08.13].

60. www.princeton.edu [Internet]. Princeton (NJ); Princeton University; Childcare assistance program for students. Available from: http://www.princeton.edu/gradschool/studentlife/childcare/sccap/; [March 8, 2012; accessed 09.08.13].

61. www.princeton.edu [Internet]. Princeton (NJ); Princeton University; Family-friendly policies and programs for Princeton faculty. Available from: http://www.princeton.edu/dof/policies/family_friendly/; [March 8, 2012; accessed 09.08.13].

62. www.princeton.edu [Internet]. Princeton (NJ); Princeton University; Family focused initiatives for graduate students. Available from: http://www.princeton.edu/gradschool/studentlife/childcare/; [March 8, 2012; accessed 09.08.13].

63. www.princeton.edu [Internet]. Princeton (NJ); Princeton University; Work life programs. Available from: http://www.princeton.edu/hr/benefits/worklife; [March 8, 2012; accessed 09.08.13].

64. uri.edu/worklife [Internet]. Kingston (RI); University of Rhode Island; Breastfeeding and lactation support program. Available from: http://www.uri.edu/worklife/_assets/Lactation%20Policy08-01FINAL.pdf; [March 8, 2012; accessed 09.08.13].

65. Silver B. College and university lactation programs [Internet]; 2010. Available from: http://www.uri.edu/worklife/family/family%20pics-docs/LactationPrograms%20FINAL.pdf; [March 8, 2012; accessed 09.08.13].

66. uri.edu/worklife [Internet]. Kingston (RI); University of Rhode Island Work-Life Resources. Available from: www.uri.edu/worklife; [March 8, 2012; accessed 09.08.13].

67. Mederer H, Silver B. *Workplace flexibility and faculty success: what a chair needs to know.* (PowerPoint presentation) Kingston (RI): University of Rhode Island Work-Life Committee; 2011. Available from: http://www.uri.edu/worklife/_assets/Resources/Presentations/Chairs'%20Work-Life%20workshop%20HM.pdf.

68. uri.edu/worklife [Internet]. Kingston (RI); University of Rhode Island Work-Life Needs Assessments; 2013. Available from: http://www.uri.edu/worklife/homepages/home%20page%20images, docs/WL%20Brkfst%20invitation.pdf, and http://www.uri.edu/worklife/survey/Survey-%20Paper%20Version-Final.pdf; [March 8, 2012; accessed 09.08.13].

69. Dean DJ. *Getting the most out of your mentoring relationships: a handbook for women in STEM*. New York: Springer, 2009.

70. Kay AC, Gaucher D, Peach JM, Laurin K, Friesen J, Zanna MP, et al. Inequality, discrimination, and the power of the status quo: direct evidence for a motivation to see the way things are as the way they should be. *J Pers Soc Psychol* September 2009;**97**(3):421–34. http://dx.doi.org/10.1037/a0015997.

71. Chambers DW. Stereotypic images of the scientist: the draw-a-scientist test. *Sci Educ* 1983;**67**(2):255–65.

72. Greenwald AG, Nosek BA, Banaji MR. Understanding and using the implicit association test: I. An improved scoring algorithm. *J Pers Soc Psychol* 2003;**85**(2):197–216.

73. Steele CM, Aronson J. Stereotype threat and the intellectual test performance of African Americans. *J Pers Soc Psychol* 1995;**69**(5):797–811.

74. Steinpreis RE, Anders KA, Ritzke D. The impact of gender on the review of the curricula vitae of job applicants and tenure candidates: a national empirical study. *Sex Roles* 1999;**41**(7–8):509–28.

75. Moss-Racusin CA, Dovidio JF, Brescoll VL, Graham MJ, Handelsman J. Science faculty's subtle gender biases favor male students. *Proc Natl Acad Sci* 2012;**109**(41):16474–9.

76. Upchurch M, Fojtová S. Women in the brain: a history of glial cell metaphors. *NWSA J* 2009;**21**(2):1–20.

77. Goldin C, Rouse C. Orchestrating impartiality: the impact of "blind" auditions on female musicians. *Am Econ Rev* 2000;**90**(4):715–41.

78. Budden AE, Tregenza T, Aarssen LW, Koricheva J, Leimu R, Lortie CJ. Double-blind review favours increased representation of female authors. *Trends Ecol Evol* 2008;**23**(1):4–6.

79. Ely RJ, Ibarra H, Kolb DM. Taking gender into account: theory and design for women's leadership development programs. *Acad Manage Learn Educ* 2011;**10**(3):474–93.

80. Isbell LA, Young TP, Harcourt AH. Stag parties linger: continued gender bias in a female-rich scientific discipline. *PLOS One* 2013;**7**(11):e49682.

81. Schroeder J, Dugdale HL, Radersma R, Hinsch M, Buehler DM, Saul J, et al. Fewer invited talks by women in evolutionary biology symposia. *J Evol Biol.* [Internet] June, 2013. Available from: http://onlinelibrary.wiley.com/doi/10.1111/jeb.12198/abstract; [accessed 09.08.13]. DOI:10.1111/jeb.12198.

82. Schmader T, Whitehead J, Wysocki VH. A linguistic comparison of letters of recommendation for male and female chemistry and biochemistry job applicants. *Sex Roles* 2007;**57**(7–8):509–14.

83. Madera JM, Hebl MR, Martin RC. Gender and letters of recommendation for academia: agentic and communal differences. *J Appl Psychol* 2009;**94**(6):1591–9.

84. Lincoln AE, Pincus S, Koster JB, Leboy PS. The Matilda effect in science: awards and prizes in the U.S., 1990s and 2000s. *Soc Stud Sci* 2012;**42**(2):307–20.

85. National Science Foundation Advance Grant #0930073. Available from: http://www.nsf.gov/awardsearch/showAward?AWD_ID=0930073&HistoricalAwards=false.

86. Popejoy A, Leboy PS. Is math still just a man's world? *J Math Syst Sci* 2013;**2**(5):292–8.

87. ilo.org [Internet]. Geneva: International Labor Organization. Available from: http://www.ilo.org/global/about-the-ilo/newsroom/news/WCMS_008009/lang–en/index.htm; [February 16, 1998; accessed 09.08.13].

88. awis.org [Internet]. Alexandria (VA): Association for Women in Science. AWIS work life survey executive summary. Available from: http://www.awis.org/associations/9417/files/AWIS_Work_Life_Balance_Executive_Summary.pdf; [March 8, 2012; accessed 09.08.13].

89. workplaceflexibility.org. [Internet]. Washington (DC): White House Forum on Workplace Flexibility. Mason MA, Goulden M, Frasch K. Keeping women in the science pipeline. Available from: http://workplaceflexibility.org/images/uploads/program_papers/mason_-_keeping_women_in_the_science_pipeline.pdf; [November 29, 2010; accessed 09.08.13].

90. bls.gov [Internet]. Washington (DC): U.S. Department of Labor, Bureau of Labor Statistics. National compensation survey: employee benefits in private industry in the United States. Available from: http://www.bls.gov/ncs/ebs/sp/ebsm0004.pdf; [August, 2006; accessed 09.08.13].

91. Kff.org. [Internet]. Menlo Park (CA): Kaiser Family Foundation. Wyn R, Ojeda V, Ranji U, Salganicoff A. Women, work and family health: a balancing act. Available from: http://kff.org/uninsured/issue-brief/women-work-and-family-health-a-balancing/; [April, 2003; accessed 09.08.13].

92. catalyst.org [Internet]. New York: Catalyst. Knowledge Center report. After-school worries: tough on parents, bad for business. Available from: http://www.catalyst.org/knowledge/after-school-worries-tough-parents-bad-business; [December 6, 2006; accessed 09.08.13].

93. nsf.gov [Internet]. Arlington (VA): National Science Foundation. Available from: http://www.nsf.gov/career-life-balance/; [September 27, 2011; updated July 2, 2013; accessed 09.08.13].

94. nih.gov [Internet]. Bethesda (MD): National Institutes of Health. Available from: http ://grants.nih.gov/grants/family_friendly.htm; [July 1, 2008; updated June 1, 2011; accessed 09.08.13].

95. uer-lex.europa.eu [Internet]. Brussels: European Union, EUR-Lex access to European Union Law. Available from: http://eur-lex.europa.eu/LexUriServ/LexUriServ.do?uri=OJ:C:2010:083:0047:0200:en:PDF; [June 2, 2013; accessed 21.09.13].

96. ec.europa.eu [Internet]. Brussels: European Commission Research Innovation. Available from: http://ec.europa.eu/research/mariecurieactions/; [August 16, 2013; accessed 21.08.13].

97. ec.europa.eu [Internet]. Brussels: European Commission. EURAXESS researchers in motion. Available from: http://ec.europa.eu/euraxess/index.cfm/rights/european Charter.

98. statcan.gc.ca [Internet]. Ottawa: Statistics Canada. Public postsecondary enrolments, by registration status, Pan-Canadian Standard Classification of Education (PCSCE), Classification of Instructional Programs, Primary Grouping (CIP_PG), sex and immigration status, 2012. Statistics Canada Table 477–0019. Available from: http://www5. statcan.gc.ca/cansim/a26?lang=eng&id=4770019&p2=17; [accessed 09.09.13].

99. Kim YO, Moon YK. *National assessments on gender and science, technology and innovation* (South Korea), Prepared for WIGSAT-OWSD ed.; 2011. Available at: http://wisat.org/data/documents/RepKorea_GE-KS.pdf.

100. Abreu A. *National assessment of gender, science, technology and innovation—Brazil qualitative report*, Prepared for WIGSAT-OWSD ed. ; 2012. Available from: http://wisat.org/data/documents/Brazil_Qual_GE-KS.pdf.

101. National Advisory Council on Innovation (NACI). *An assessment of the participation of women in science, engineering and technology industry*; 2008. Pretoria. (Report commissioned by the South African Reference Group on Women in Science and Technology (SARG)).

102. statcan.gc.ca [Internet]. Ottawa: Statistics Canada. Employment by industry and sex. Available from: http://www.statcan.gc.ca/tables-tableaux/sum-som/l01/cst01/labor10a-eng.htm; [2012; accessed 09.09.13].

103. Council of Canadian Academies. Strengthening Canada's research capacity: the gender dimension. The Expert Panel on Women in University Research, ed. Ottawa: Council of Canadian Academies, 2012. Available from: http://www.scienceadvice.ca/uploads/eng/assessments%20and%20publications%20and%20news%20releases/Women_University_Research/WUR_fullreportEN.pdf.pdf.

104. World Bank. *World development report 2012: Gender equality and development*. Washington, DC: World Bank; 2012. Available from: http://econ.worldbank.org/WBSITE/EXTERNAL/EXTDEC/EXTRESEARCH/EXTWDRS/EXTWDR2012/0,contentMDK:22999750~menuPK:8154981~pagePK:64167689~piPK:64167673~theSitePK:7778063,00.html.

105. Oliveira MC, Marcondes GS, Viera JM, Aparicio R. *National assessments on gender and STI – Brazil.* Women in Global Science and Technology (WISAT), Organization for Women in Science for the Developing World (OWSD); 2011. Available from: http://wisat.org/data/documents/Brazil_Quant_GE-KS.pdf.

106. Central Statistics Office. *Women and men in India.* 13th issue ed. New Delhi: Ministry of Statistics and Programme Implementation, Government of India; 2011. Available from: http://mospi.nic.in/Mospi_New/upload/women_men_2011_31oct11.pdf.

107. Nair S. *National assessment of the participation of women and girls in the National STI system based on the gender equality-knowledge society framework,* Prepared for WIGSAT-owsd; 2011. Available from: http://wisat.org/data/documents/India_GE-KS.pdf.

108. Department of Science and Technology. Evaluating and enhancing women's participation in S&T research: the Indian initiatives. Report of the national Task Force for women in science ed. New Delhi: Ministry of science and Technology, Government of India, 2009.

109. Fortin P, Godbut L, St-Cerny S. Economic consequences of Quebec's educational childcare policy. Paper presented at the Early Years Economics Forum. June 22, 2011, Toronto (ON). ed. 2011. Available from: http://www.mwmccain.ca/media/uploads/does-preschool-education-pay/EarlyLearningEconomicForum_Fortin.pdf.

110. Heylman SR. South Korea plans flexible work system for government workers. SHRM Knowledge Centre. Society for Human Resource Management. Available from: http://www.shrmindia.org/knowledge-center/employee-relationship/workplace-flexibility/south-korea-plans-flexible-work-system-government-workers; [March 24, 2010; accessed 16.09.13].

111. balita.ph [Internet]. Glendale (CA): The Balita Organization. Only 10 percent of Korean firms adopt flexible work system. Balita. Available from: http://balita.ph/2013/05/08/only-10-percent-of-korean-firms-adopt-flexible-work-system/; [May 8, 2013; accessed 06.09.13].

112. Singh N, Sinha P. RBI offers its officers flexible work timings. *The Times of India.* Available from: http://articles.timesofindia.indiatimes.com/2013-04-02/india-business/38216734_1_rbi-office-the-rbi-alpana-killawala; [April 2, 2013; accessed 06.09.13].

113. southasia.oneworld.net [Internet]. Rahman, AP. For women in India, flexi-time translates into productive work. One World South Asia. Available from: http://southasia.oneworld.net/features/india-for-women-flexi-time-translates-into-productive-work#; UiobTOBYRkE. [July 19, 2013; accessed 06.09.13].

114. Lee, KJB. Effective policies for supporting education and employment of women in science and technology. United Nations Commission for the Status of Women Expert paper prepared for the expert group meeting on gender, science and technology, Available from: http://www.un.org/womenwatch/daw/egm/gst_2010/Lee-EP.6-EGM-ST.pdf; September 28–October 1, 2010.

Index

Note: Page numbers followed by "f" denote figures; "t" tables.

Printed and bound by CPI Group (UK) Ltd, Croydon, CR0 4YY

03/10/2024

01040420-0002